The Chinese Art of
T'AI CHI CH'UAN

A dynamic aid to health and inner tranquillity
through controlled movements for self-defence
and the development of physical and mental powers.

D0109991

By the same author:
THE TAO OF LONG LIFE
TAOIST ART OF FENG SHOU
TAOIST YOGA

The Chinese Art of
T'AI CHI CH'UAN

by
CHEE SOO

THE AQUARIAN PRESS
Wellingborough, Northamptonshire

First published 1984
Fourth Impression 1985

British Library Cataloguing in Publication Data

Soo, Chee
    T'ai chi ch'uan: the Taoist way to mental
    and physical health.
    1. T'ai chi ch'uan
    I. Title
    613.7'1   GV505

    ISBN 0-85030-387-7

*The Aquarian Press is part of the
Thorsons Publishing Group*

Printed and bound in Great Britain

To Marilyn

My sincere gratitude for everything
you have done — thank you.

Contents

Preface

T'iyu (Taoist Physical Culture) has been handed down for over 10,000 years. For the last 3,000 years the Lee family has been responsible for handing down these arts, and it is a wonderful honour to pass on their intimate knowledge to you.

Because the Lee family Taoists arts were never put into print, it gives me great pleasure to present this introduction to the Lee family style of the Taoist art of T'ai Chi Ch'uan, which is also the only 'Yin and Yang' style in the world.

T'ai Chi Ch'uan has proved, over and over again, to be one of the finest ways of improving health, assisting the flow of the circulation of blood, creating tranquility throughout the entire nervous system, and through the concentration it requires, creating a deep peace of mind. Through the harmony of mind and body comes great happiness and good health.

Our T'ai Chi Ch'uan style is also sometimes referred to as the 'Square Yard T'ai Chi', because all the movements can be performed within a square yard of floor space, which enables everyone to practise daily in their own home without having to move the furniture.

No matter where you go, you will find that the people who practise our style are wonderful, and we all make a lot of friends no matter where we go. It's a true family style, so we welcome you to join our family of thousands throughout the world, and learn the depths of the 'Supreme Ultimate,' for we are the only association that teaches the true depths of yourself within the form of T'ai Chi Ch'uan.

CHEE SOO

Chapter 1

The History of T'ai Chi Ch'uan

When they first see a demonstration of T'ai Chi Ch'uan (The Supreme Ultimate) most people are fascinated by the beauty of the performer's movements, and naturally assume that it comprises a sequence of physical callisthenics. This is only partly true although it did have its very early beginnings in the various forms of pugilism that existed in China for many thousands of years.

In very ancient China, superstition, divination, spiritualism, and religion went through various stages of development and advancement, and played a very important part in everyday life. The roofs of Chinese houses were turned up at the eaves so that the dragon could rest on its travels through the sky, and it could even curl up and go to sleep without falling off the end of the roof. Even the dead had to be buried in exactly the right position, so that their spirit would not be hindered in its flight from the grave, and every village had its own specialist to advise bereaved families how and where their dead should be buried.

There were many different aspects of divination and spiritualism that had to be studied, and theories that had to be proved. These all provided a very valuable foundation for the development of codes of thought and mental conduct, the discovery of the fundamental workings of the body, the discovery of the harmony that existed within the universe, and the exploration of the depths of the spiritual world.

The goals of immortality and a longer life included the search for constant good health, a greater understanding and control of oneself, the full utilization of the mind, and a greater appreciation of the world beyond the physical aspects of the human body.

Taoism came into being in China between 10,000 and 5,000 BC, and it was through the dedication and hard work of the early Taoists that they were able to develop so many arts and crafts from the foundations and guidelines given to them by the 'Sons of Reflected Light', a sect of people reputed to be over seven feet in height, and who wore a type of clothing that had never been seen in China before. Where they came from is still a mystery, and may remain a mystery for ever, but whilst they stayed they taught local craftspeople many different arts and crafts, which were far in advance of anything else that existed in those far off days. Many of these skills are still in advance of anything that is in existence even in this present day and age.

Great efforts have been made by the Taoists through the ages to carry on this good work and to pass on the knowledge that was given to them by the 'Sons of Reflected Light'. Unfortunately, since no written records were kept in those far distant days, some of their teachings have no doubt been lost in the realms of time.

Amongst the skills that were passed on are silk-weaving, glass and pottery making, the manufacture of gun-powder, and metal working. The most important of all, however, is the vast array of health skills, many of which are still being practised and taught today.

These health arts eventually became known as the 'Eight Strands of the Brocade' (Pa Chin Hsien), and in the West they are still being used to help sufferers of all types of disease and infirmity, often completely free of charge. This philosophical outlook is still carried on within Taoist families, for when it is your birthday you give your parents and your brothers and sisters a present each to thank them and to show your appreciation of being brought into this world amongst such nice people. We still keep up this practise in our house.

The 'Eight Strands of the Brocade' comprise eight distinct sections of the health arts:

1. Chen Tuan — Diagnosis
2. Ch'ang Ming — Natural Health Therapy

3. Ts'ao Yao   — Herbal Therapy
4. Wen Chiech'u   — Contact Thermogenesis
5. Hsia Chen Pien — Acupuncture
6. Tien An   — Acupressure
7. Anmo (T'ui Na) — Massage
8. Ch'ili Nung   — The Way of Occlusion

All these arts have been kept alive by the Taoists for many thousands of years. They aimed for two major objectives: to maintain a longer life here on this earth, and to achieve a stronger spiritual link with the Supreme Spirit. They endeavoured to achieve these aims by accepting each day and event as it came along, by understanding and abiding by the infinite laws of the universe and of the Tao. This consciousness and awareness gives a deep appreciation of the physical, mental and energy (Chi) aspects of the human body. It also gives a perfect balance of Yin and Yang by helping each person to appreciate the spiritual side of their lives, of the Tao, and of the energy fields within the universe (Li). All of these keep us alive, maintain our health, and guide every day of our lives.

Many people see the physical side of our lives as separate from our spiritual life, but this is not true, for the two sides represent Yin and Yang. In both East and West there are many groups who have believed in the spiritual side more than their bodily development, and many who have only considered the physical aspect. These varying trends of thought have affected and infiltrated into the major forms of T'ai Chi Ch'uan. Today there are only three well-known styles of this art in existence. One of these, the Wu style, has almost disappeared.

The Wu Style
The originator of this particular style was a gentleman by the name of Yu-Seong Wu, and he studied T'ai Chi when he was in his early twenties, in the Province of Honan. However, when he was in his late fifties he created a completely new style of his own, which consisted of very small circular movements, short arm flow, and rather restricted stances. It came into being during the eighteenth century, but has never been really popular nor very well known. Some years ago we heard that there was still one school in Hong Kong still practising it, but we have heard nothing about it since

then, so it is quite possible that is has ceased to function. It was apparently a very difficult style to follow even on a physical level, and the energy required was minimal, as most of the movements were neutralized.

The Yang Style

Lu-Ch'an Yang is recognized as the founder of this particular style which became firmly established between 1883 and 1936, when Ch'eng-fu Yang (Yang's grandson) became the chief instructor of this style and opened his own school. Lu-Ch'an Yang himself first became interested in T'ai Chi when he had the opportunity of studying the Ch'en style, which alas no longer exists today. This Yang style has been altered and improved three times since it first came into existence. Twice Lu-Ch'an Yang changed and incorporated his own personal ideas into the old Ch'en style he originally learnt, and it again went through some slight alterations after Ch'eng-fu Yang opened his T'ai Chi school in 1883.

The movements of this particular style are large and rhythmic, and it flows with varying fluctuations of light and heavy techniques. It is a very popular style wherever it is taught, for it is generally recognized as the form for those who like to be physical and who are interested in fighting and boxing.

The Lee Style

The Lee style is commonly known as the Yin and Yang Style, as everything within it is in complete harmony and in perfect balance with each other. It is the only true Taoist art, the oldest form of T'ai Chi Ch'uan in existence, and the most popular style in the world.

Up to 1934 it had always remained a family style, and it was originally created by Ho-Hsieh Lee around 1,000 BC, so this style is nearly three thousand years old. The original form consisted only of eight movements, and those same movements still exist within the form as it is today, which now comprises a total of 140 single movements, in the form of forty-two sets.

Originally Ho-Hsieh Lee and his family lived just outside Beijing (Peking), and it was there that he first started his practise and devised the first eight movements. It was in his middle fifties that he took his family and settled down in Wei Hei Wei, a fishing village about 200 miles east of Beijing, and they remained in that district up to 1934.

The family had always been Taoists and had practised the Chinese Taoist arts, including Feng Shou Ch'uan Shu (Hand-of-the-Wind Boxing); Ch'i Shu (Energy Art), the equivalent of Chinese Aikidi; Chiao Li (Taoist Wrestling); and the complete range of T'ai Chi Ch'uan — T'ai Chi Stick, T'ai Chi Sword, T'ai Chi Knife, and more recently T'ai Chi Dance.

As it was a family group and they practised together, it was natural that the parents instructed their children, who in turn taught their own children, and so on. Thus it came about that the last three children, one daughter and two sons, had the responsibility of keeping the arts alive. In fact only one son did so, and his name was Chan Kam Lee, the eldest of the three children.

Chan Lee, an unmarried businessman dealing in precious and semi-precious stones, finally opened a small office in the Holborn district of London, which in those days was the world centre of this trade. In 1933 he started a small class in Red Lion Square, Holborn, to keep himself fit and to benefit a few selected close friends.

I was playing in Hyde Park with my ball one Sunday afternoon in 1934, and I remember that my ball accidentally hit the back of an elderly gentleman who was sitting on a park bench. Offering my sincere apologies to him, we noticed that both of us were Chinese, and we immediately started talking to one another, since it was a rarity to see another Chinese in London in those days. A bond of friendship immediately sprang up between the two of us, and I was eventually invited to join his little group in Holborn.

In the winter of 1953/4 Chan Kam Lee died in a severe storm off the coast of China near Canton, and eventually I was asked to take over as Chief Instructor and President of the Association.

To me it has been the greatest honour to carry on the work of the Lee family. It will always be known as the Lee style, and regular coaching classes are held in many parts of the world to ensure that we are all teaching and practising the movements and techniques as specifically laid down by the Lee family. The names of the postures or stances still use the names of animals and birds which were used three thousand years ago. The Lee style has been preserved through many centuries, and we all hope that it will continue to flourish and grow for many more.

Chapter 2

The Principles of
the Supreme Ultimate

Why should this beautiful sequence of movements be known as the 'Supreme Ultimate' (T'ai Chi)? Does it mean that we have to achieve absolute perfection in every movement that we execute, or does it mean that we are aiming for an ultimate goal in everything which is a true component of this wonderful art?

There are thousands of people in the West who have gained great benefit from the practise of T'ai Chi Ch'uan, and there are many more who are seriously interested in learning. Unfortunately many of these people learn only the physical aspect of the form, and therefore gain very little from it. Many of them spend a great deal of time in practice, yet without discovering the full depth and potential of the art, all their work is doing no more than scratching the surface. Even their physical progress is limited, because the most important depths of their physical selves remain unused and undiscovered.

The majority of T'ai Chi schools teach only the physical side of the whole art. They sincerely believe that they are progressing by just learning the stances, but inwardly they are often doing more harm than good, because by remaining on a physical level they never express their complete selves, and in so doing retard their own progress in the wholeness of life.

This is a shame, for after setting themselves to learn the art over a long period of time, practising for many hours and showing great interest and dedication, their efforts have often been completely wasted. They have not progressed at all on the physical level, and have never learnt the other dynamic aspects of this wonderful art.

The truth is that there are five complete sections in the complete training of T'ai Chi Ch'uan, so every student should ensure that they train under the supervision of a fully qualified teacher who can not only teach these five sections but can also demonstrate them. Then and only then will the student gain maximum benefit from this art in every respect, have a complete understanding of its true depth, and develop an awareness which they had not previously known existed.

The Lee style is taught through the auspices of the International Taoist Society, who are ensuring that the Taoist Arts, which were maintained and developed by the Lee family, will always remain exactly as they wanted them to be. The Society also ensures that this great depth of knowledge will only be taught by teachers who have qualified, practised, and been taught within the Society.

Let us now look at the five sections of T'ai Chi Ch'uan as taught by the International Taoist Society.

1. The Physical

The first step is to ensure that you are eating and drinking sensibly, and it is recommended that anyone who is seriously interested in permanent good health should try to adhere to the rules laid down by the early Taoists. These are called Ch'ang Ming (The Taoist Health Therapy for a long Healthy Life).

The second step is to start to practise the various physical aspects of the sections of the 'form' by aiming towards perfection of the stances (legs), posture (body) and technique (hands and arms). Having learnt a few movements or sections, try to magnify your sensitivity by learning to feel the rhythm and flow within the technique of your hands and arms, and match and harmonize the rhythm and flow from one stance of your legs and feet to another. Be dedicated and practise a few movements daily, morning and evening, and you will eventually achieve these aims.

Remember, whilst you will be utilizing your body to evaluate the depths of your movements, you must never become solely physical, or try to use your strength, for by so doing you will restrict your own development.

Many T'ai Chi teachers will tell you that your movements will exercise the whole body. In fact the parts of the body are complementary — it is the top that exercises the bottom and the bottom the top. The right exercises the left and the left the right. In our arts we prove this to you in a multiplicity of ways, so you learn to appreciate and understand your own body even more. Total harmony and perfection of all the movements is essential to achieve the ultimate of your physical self.

2. The Mental

From the very beginning of your physical practise you will find that you become more mentally active, and a great deal of concentration is required to obtain the perfection you are aiming for and your teacher expects. You have to harmonize your stance on both left and right legs, attain the correct angle of your whole body, top and bottom and right and left. Then there are all the variations in your hands and arms, which can move in totally different directions, create their own characteristics, and move at varying speeds. All this is created by the mind, and must all be controlled from the mental source. A simple act of emptying the mind, as some try to do in meditation, actually fills it, so that it becomes more active than ever.

Dynamic mental control can create a tranquil mind without its being empty. It can utilize power without the use of strength, cause heaviness without weight, create length from shortness and speed from slowness.

All these aspects of mental control are practised continuously in all our Taoist arts classes. Perhaps one day you too will be able to execute every movement of T'ai Chi Ch'uan by remaining absolutely stationary and immobile. When you reach this very advanced stage, you can go one step further by practising the various aspects of the Taoist Wand (Taoist Mokun), which is the advanced control of energies by the mind.

3. Breathing

Most people breathe in and out every minute of every day and never give it a second thought, unless they have some sort of respiration problem. Yet the Taoists of ancient China created over fifty different specialized breathing exercises, all of which are incorporated into our arts in a special section called Hu Hsi Ichih (Taoist Respiration Therapy). Amongst them are many special breathing techniques which also incorporate specific physical exercises, purposely designed to assist in the cure of many different illnesses connected to specific organs of the body.

In addition to these, there are other very special breathing exercises that help to activate or sedate the natural energy (Sheng Chi) of the body, and these exercises are an integral part of our training.

It is important for a beginner to take things easy at the beginning of their training. Very few people have learnt to breathe fully, so their bodies are not used to dealing with a large amount of oxygen. Even fewer people have learnt to breathe deeply in the lower abdomen (Tan Tien). Thus in the early stages of learning the form let your breathing be as natural as possible, then slowly your teacher will help you to co-ordinate your breathing with your movements and your mind.

If your breathing remains natural, then slowly through your training you will be able to let it sink lower and lower until it eventually reaches the lower abdomen. Your early training will also assist in this matter, because through correct stances with relaxed bodies and relaxed movements, breathing will naturally sink lower. Once breathing into the lower abdomen becomes natural and automatic, the energy of the body (Sheng Chi) will be enhanced.

4. Sheng Chi

The development of natural energy is dependent on eating and drinking the Ch'ang Ming way, so that the tissues of the body become more supple and flexible, thereby helping the body to accept really deep breathing. Really deep breathing should take place in the lower abdomen, because this is where there are two energy centres, one of which is where the Chi develops and stores itself. As coal is the fuel of a fire, so breath is the fuel of the natural energy of the body. Respiration exercises are thus a natural part of Chi development. Sheng Chi (Vitality Power) was also called 'Internal Energy' (Nei Pu Chi) or 'Intrinsic Energy' (T'ien Jan Neng Li), and it is the energy that everyone who practises our Taoist arts strives to cultivate.

A strong Chi helps everyone to attain permanent good health. In our Taoist arts we learn to use it whilst practising our form of T'ai Chi Ch'uan, and learn also how we use it in every part of our lives, whether at work or at play.

Its force is colossal and far greater than brute strength can ever be, enabling anybody — man or woman — to have the power of five people. The amazing thing about it is that you were born with it, and you possess it all your lives. Its benefit to your health is beyond the understanding of the average person, but it helps to fight germs and bacteria within the human body, and a truly strong Chi will improve your health to such a degree that colds and influenza are never experienced.

The Chi is invisible, it has no aroma, and you cannot hear it, yet it is an integral part of your body and it influences your daily life. It is substantial and insubstantial; it is unyielding yet pliability itself; it is soft and gentle yet it can be as hard as steel; it is weightless yet it cannot be lifted. Our arts teach us to know what it is, and where it is stored and generated, and how we can cultivate, utilize and control it. When your health is really good and you have practised our arts for some time, then you will be able to feel the flow of your own Chi through your body.

Like mental energy, Sheng Chi depends for its strength and regeneration on the personal good health of the person, constant deep breathing, and relaxation. That is why T'ai Chi Ch'uan is good for the health in so many different ways. We must be able to store energy before we can use it, and we must learn to conserve our vitality before we can achieve good health.

Most people in the West, particularly those who live or work in cities, find it very difficult to relax, and require additional aids to help them to do so. The Taoist art of T'ai Chi Ch'uan has the answer. Besides the specialized warming up exercises which all our classes commence with, there are also a number of simple breathing exercises that help to develop this vital energy.

Here is a simple breathing exercise that you might like to try. Begin by sitting on a chair or, preferably, cross-legged (your left leg outside your right) on the floor, freeing your body and mind from outside influences and internal tensions. Place your hands flat on your abdomen, and whilst keeping your body fairly upright without stiffness, allow your shoulders to drop as low as they will go. You may notice that your chest will depress slightly, but don't worry about it, it is quite natural.

Now take a deep inward breath (Chi Hsi) through the nose, but instead of letting the air fill your lungs and chest, allow your breath to sink so that your abdomen swells outward. Then exhale

(Hu Chi) through the nose, but as you do so, press your hands firmly against the abdomen, so that you force the stale air out through your nostrils. Repeat this sequence six times daily. Whenever you feel tired and run down, use this breathing exercise. By repeating it regularly, your health will benefit and you will feel better within yourself.

It takes the average person in the West about six months to a year to begin to feel the vitality power within themselves. Once having learnt to feel this energy, the next step is to direct it from the lower abdomen to any other part of the body through mental control.

This is known as 'propelled movement' (T'uichin Kutung), and it is only by obtaining mastery of it that a person can attain true mastery of their own energies.

5. Ching Sheng Li

This energy is known as 'macro-cosmic' or 'external' energy. It is the natural energy of the universe, for it comes down from the heavens, passes through everything on this earth, including our own bodies, enters the earth and, after gathering further vitality and power, returns upwards to return from whence it came. It is constantly present and passing through our human bodies, and it can be harnessed, stored, controlled and utilized by everyone, providing they have the mental training to do so.

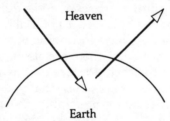

Heaven

Earth

By utilizing this dynamic energy, many ancient Chinese philosophers lived from 150 to 200 years of age, and even in this modern era it is possible to have, even at the age of sixty, the skin, body, mentality, energy and vitality of a twenty-year-old. It is not time or the number of years that matter, it is the true health of the individual that eventually shows through. The Taoist will tell you and show you the real truth: keeping fit does not necessarily make you truly healthy, but if you are truly healthy then you are automatically fit.

On its downward journey Ching Sheng Li passes through all men, down the spine and out through the lower abdomen. This circular action is centripetal in its flow, and this Li energy moves in this way through all Yang things. On its upward path, or return journey from the earth, it passes through everything that is Yin, in a centrifugal motion. In passing through all women it comes up from the ground, along the spine, and out through the head. These two directions are represented as follows:

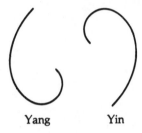

Yang   Yin

When these two directions were placed together by the ancient Taoists, they represented the well-known Yin and Yang symbol:

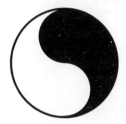

Not only did this concept represent Yin and Yang, showing the two sides of everything, but it also expressed the idea that nothing had a beginning nor an end, everything is everlasting. Later, the ancient Taoists added a further permutation, as you will see in the next chapter, which demonstrated their closer appreciation of the work of the Tao.

A more complex symbolic expression of the workings of the universe is the Eight Trigrams (Pa Kua) which are included in the *Book of Changes (I Ching)*, which is one of the most important books in the world, for thousands of years of wisdom and understanding have gone into it. Both Confucianism and Taoism have their roots here, so it is natural that the basic principles of T'ai Chi Ch'uan are derived from it.

Chapter 3

Yin and Yang

The Lee family 'Yin and Yang' style of T'ai Chi Ch'uan will enable every student to obtain the full benefits of every aspect of the art, and they will also obtain a complete understanding of its great depth and wonderful harmony with all things within the universe.

It will help to develop dynamic mental control over the physical aspects of the body as well as the superb handling of the energies, and it will not only greatly increase the complete utilization of everything within us, but it will help us to acquire a perfect balance. In its own way, it will also help us to attain a greater spiritual awareness and understanding. Naturally, the underlying Taoist philosophy helps to make it a way of life, and all those who practise it strive to become one with themselves and eventually one with nature. In this way, T'ai Chi Ch'uan can be of enormous benefit to all those who practise it with sincere dedication.

The foundations of the understanding of T'ai Chi Ch'uan — the 'Supreme Ultimate' or 'Great Ultimate', or (as it is now called in China) the 'Great Extreme' or the 'Great Ridgepole' — are the very simple principles of Yin and Yang, which express the monism and dualism, the singular and plural, the unity and opposition of everything in nature, within our own lives and within our spirits.

We are all one with the Supreme Spirit, yet, at the same time, we still remain our own individual self, so through a very natural principle an automatic duality is created. This duality also applies to everything within the universe, for everything has two sides, a positive and a negative, a back and a front, a top and a bottom. At the same time everything is one within itself, and has its own Yin and Yang relationship. The being one is known as monism; the natural diversity which has been created by the universe gives everything a balance of two as well: this is dualism, Yin and Yang. Because of this simple arrangement, the combination of the two ideas, dual-monism, covers the whole as well as the singular.

Nothing could be more simple than monism within everything, yet the complexity of dualism can often be beyond the imaginations of the mind. By taking things step by step, you will slowly appreciate and understand the various aspects of every single object, and then and only then will the dualist view of everything be made known to you.

Before the universe came into existence there was the void, and from it came the macro-cosmic energy known as Ching Sheng Li. At the very beginning of time, this force divided into two parts under the strict control of the Supreme Spirit, and this duality came to be known as the Yin and Yang. It was after this division that the energy created substance, and so heaven and earth eventually became reality.

The Yin aspect represents the body, soul, femininity, earth, moon, night, darkness, cold, water, contraction and centripetal motion, and has the tendency to flow downwards. Yang, on the other hand, has characteristics that are completely opposite: mind, spirit, masculinity, sun, day, fire, heat, expansion, centrifugal motion and an upward direction of flow. One very important thing to notice is that nothing is entirely Yin or entirely Yang, for where there is the one there will always be a small part of the other.

Never make the mistake of thinking that everything can be classed as totally Yin or Yang, as this would be wrong. Nothing is absolute. These are general tendencies, and they represent differences between all phenomena that exist within the universe. That is why the ancient Chinese Taoists represented the balance of the two through the flow of energy within ourselves as:

This shows very clearly that within the one there is always a certain amount of the other.

The monad or monism which is associated with Yin concentrates on the one and the unity of all things, within the universe and within ourselves. The duad or dualism is connected with Yang and it automatically recognizes the diversity and duality within all things. For example, a coin could be thought of as Yin, but because a true coin has two sides — a head and a tail — it is also Yang in contrast. There is always a harmony of one with two, of singular with plural, of monism with dualism.

Dual-monism comprehends the separateness and yet the unity of all things. Since we know that nothing is entirely Yin or Yang, but a combination of both, when the two are combined entirely together we have the complete vision, the total perception, the combined harmony and the full understanding. In the recognition of this harmony we can appreciate the contrasts of Yin and Yang, and the changes that take place within nature.

All things move to infinity, but are still infinitesimal. Yet being infinitesimal they pertain to the infinite. Whilst they may be separate they are still one, yet in their separation they are completely harmonized.

In the Taoist arts both monism and dualism are symbolized by triangles, the one being an inversion of the other. The universe is symbolized by a circle, and this is seen as embracing the Yin and Yang within all things:

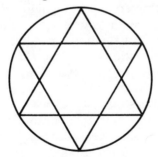

This symbol stands for everything within and outside the cosmos — heaven and earth, nature and humanity, and all phenomena both known and yet undiscovered. All are one — this is the Tao.

The positive understanding of Yin and Yang gave the ancient Taoists a very deep insight into the vibrations and strength of energy from various types of food, but only through thousands of years of constant experimentation was full knowledge eventually gained. As a result of this fantastic dedication they found the way to attain a perfect balance in their eating habits, and as a result Ch'ang Ming (Taoist Good Health and Long Life Therapy) came into being. It is still being carried on today, thanks to the work of the Lee family over the last few thousand years, and particularly to Chan Lee, who showed how the Taoist Ch'ang Ming could be adapted to Western eating habits.

As a result, Ch'ang Ming is now available to all who want to obtain the correct balance of Yin and Yang in their own bodies, to attain constant good health, and so greatly increase their chances of longevity.

The duality of the Yin and Yang is very evident in the human body, for the viscera are Yin whilst the bowel system is Yang; the exterior of the body is Yang whilst the interior is Yin; the right side of the body is Yang and the left side is Yin, and so on. There is no escaping these very simple laws within ourselves, and to attain true harmony within ourselves we must achieve a correct balance at all times. That is why a Ch'ang Ming diet is a necessity for all those who are seriously interested in their own welfare and good health.

T'ai Chi Ch'uan also has this common link with good health, for the Lee family style is a perfect balance of Yin and Yang through its stances, postures, hand movements, breathing and the essences of the energies which everyone is taught to use. It aims to achieve the Supreme Ultimate within ourselves through the processes of awakening, awareness, activation and cultivation of the vitalities and energies that are within our body. T'ai Chi Ch'uan also has a very strong link with Taoist Yoga (K'ai Men), and this is why they are invariably taught within the same class. Both aim for the Supreme Ultimate, so whilst they may travel different roads, they both have the same objective, the unification of everything within and outside of ourselves, according to the universal laws of Yin and Yang.

Chapter 4

The Aims Towards Perfection

The author of this book has been practising T'ai Chi Ch'uan for fifty years, and knows deep down inside that even though others may think what you do is perfect, something you feel and appreciate can continue to be understood ever more deeply as time goes on. Yes, perfection is a word that has no boundaries, for only you can fix the limit of yourself. However, from my own personal experience and from the foundations created by my own master, let me pass on a few tips that will help you in your training and practise, because your teacher cannot watch or be near you all the time during your endless search to become better and better.

The Supreme Ultimate
For the truly dedicated person this is the ultimate goal pointed out to us by the Taoists of ancient China, and from my own personal experience I know it is true. In simple words, it means the complete understanding, harmony and conquering of our body, mind, spirit, our own Chi energy and universal Li energy.

The Body
You will learn in the International Taoist Society that every movement has a meaning, every meaning contains a depth, and each depth contains an essence, and through the full utilization of the essence, you will find out the true meaning of the expressions that our old masters told us. Thus you will prove to yourself that 'the weakest is the strongest', 'the lightest is the heaviest', and 'the

shortest is the longest'. You will recognize these truths over and over again, until you are fully aware of the essence they contain, and how they can be utilized not only in our arts, but in your everyday life.

The first golden rule is to let your body remain relaxed and natural at all times, without any tension whatsoever. But relaxation does not mean giving way completely and slumping as if you were a dead weight. It means being your natural self, without being artificial or going to the other extreme of trying to be too precise. T'ai Chi is therapeutic, for it gives very gentle exercise to all parts of the body. When you move the arms you exercise the legs, and when you activate the legs then you automatically exercise the upper parts of your body. So harmony within all movements is very important, and co-ordination between the upper limbs and lower extremities is an important aim towards perfection.

The Legs
The legs are used to support the weight of your body at all times, and even when you are lying down muscle changes take place through the legs as the body turns. The legs, therefore, play an important part in all movements of the torso, so never oppose these natural dynamics of your own body. Other styles of T'ai Chi have quite large stances, with their body weight supported between the two legs with both knees bent. This, you will be told, conforms to the laws of gravity.

In a physical and materialistic sense they are right. We, on the other hand, explore the true meaning of the 'Supreme Ultimate' by using the essences that our legs can give, so you will find if you train with us that our weight distribution is changed for each particular stance, for this is essential to bring out the true essence that it contains. For instance, it is a golden rule in our T'ai Chi that when the foot is moved, the heel is placed on the floor first, then the ball of the foot, and finally the toes, just as if you were walking naturally. This movement from heel to toe is performed no matter what the angle of the foot might be, whether you step forward, back, or sideways, and even when you walk the air. This is not easy at first, so constant practise is recommended in order to maintain your balance while keeping control of your leg movements, which you should practise very slowly and lightly.

Learn to move from one leg movement to another, and ensure that you check and correct them constantly. Using a full length mirror is an excellent way to correct yourself.

The Arms and Hands

Never fully straighten the arms, but always keep them slightly bent. Keep your elbows pointing down, except on the rare occasions when the arms are raised above head height. Ensure that your arms are completely relaxed, irrespective of how they are moved or held.

The hand movements not only have a meaning in their flow from one direction to another, but there is a far greater depth and meaning within the essence that they contain. Perfection in the execution of the movements of hands and arms is very important indeed. There is a wise saying within our Taoist arts: 'the slowest is the fastest'. One illustration of this is a learner driver, who, once having mastered the techniques of driving very slowly, may well gain sufficient experience one day to become a champion racing driver. This applies to our arts as well. Don't rush, give yourself time to perfect a movement, harmonize it with your posture, stance and breathing, and feel the essence that it contains. Then and only then will you have acquired the mental control to harmonize every aspect in one beautiful technique — at any speed you wish.

The hands are very important, but in our everyday life we are apt to take them for granted, and never really give them a second thought unless we injure them, in which case we feel very lost. They are also extremely important in T'ai Chi, because of the intricate movements and patterns they have to execute. Complete control over them is essential at all times, whether they are moving, stationary, open or closed into a fist. There are seven main types of hand formations.

The first is the Sun Palm (Jih Shouchang). The hand is pushed forward with the fingers completely relaxed, but pointing upwards. In this formation the vitality power flows from the lower abdomen (Tan Tien) up the spine, down the arm and into the palm. This movement of the hand and arm looks very soft and gentle, but the force pushed out of the Sun Palm, with mental control, is quite dynamic.

The second is the Cloudy Palm (Yun Shouchang). The back

of the hand faces away from you and the palm is turned inward, fingers pointing upwards. The vitality power is recalled back to the lower abdomen. The hands and arms are completely relaxed and the shoulders are allowed to sink.

The third is the Crane's Head Palm (Hao T'ou Shouchang). The fingers point downwards. The shoulders, arms and hands are now completely relaxed and loose, with the vitality power having been recalled back to the lower abdomen.

The fourth is the Lifting Palm (Chu Ch'i Shouchang). The back of the hand faces the floor and the palm faces upward. The vitality power may or may not be activated, whichever you decide.

The fifth is the Side Palm (Pien Shouchang). The tip of the thumb points upwards, and the edge of the little finger downwards. In this formation the vitality power will remain stationary unless you wish to activate it through your mental control.

The sixth is the Hammer Palm (Ch'ui Shouchang). The hand is firm, the palm faces downwards, and the little finger edge would, if required, become the striking edge. The vitality power flows very forcefully into the hand, especially to the little finger edge.

The seventh is the Closed Palm, or fist (Kuan Shouchang). The fingers are closed into the palm but should remain fairly loose. The vitality power in this formation is rather restricted.

The Head and Neck
Some say that you should imagine your head being suspended, but if you do then you become like a puppet, light headed and floating. So don't let your head and neck be stiff, like that of a robot; just keep them both naturally upright, without any tension, and align them both with your spine. One day you will be amazed at the depth of essence they contain.

Breathing
Breath is life, as we all know, but correct breathing is even more important than that. Not only does it sustain life and purify the blood, but it is also the fuel for the vitality energy of the body, just as coal is fuel for a fire.

In your early days of training, however, we suggest that you shouldn't worry too much about breathing. If you join one of our affiliated clubs or classes you will be taught many specialized breathing exercises, but for the beginner who practises at home without an instructor, we suggest that you first practise some of the sequences over and over again. This will enable you to attain the perfection of stances and postures and a continuous flow of movement, and during these early periods you should just breathe naturally through the nose as you practise.

As all movements of our T'ai Chi Ch'uan style are based on an in-and-out movement, breathing can easily be harmonized with them. On the odd numbers or inward movements you should breathe in, and on the even numbers or outward movements you should breathe out. Your health will feel the benefit, and you will gradually learn to take deeper and longer breaths as you learn to co-ordinate the length of your inhalations and exhalations with your movements.

Next, try and learn to breathe in through the nose and out through the mouth when practising the movements, and time them to your breathing, rather than timing your breathing to your movements.

The next stage is to learn to breathe deeply into the area below your navel. Lower abdominal breathing (Tan T'ien Ch'i Hsi) not only excites and activates the vitality power, but it also helps to give you an internal massage by the expansion and contraction of the muscles and the intestines. It helps to improve blood circulation and liver functions and generally aids the working of the body metabolism. At first you will have to concentrate the mind on the sinking of the breath down to the Tan Tien. In Taoist thought and Chinese alchemy, the lower abdomen is known as the 'lower cauldron', and it can only be reached and activated by deep diaphragmatic breathing (what the Taoists call Yang breathing).

The Tan Tien is also a psychic centre of primary importance, and the main centre for the storage and circulation of Chi and Li energies. The harmonious mixture of Chi and Li energies in the lower abdomen is known in Taoist thought as 'the Inner Circle'. The same area also acts as the centre of the 'Outer Circle' of the body, which governs the spiritual and psychic channels of the mind and body. It must therefore be looked after, nurtured and protected, for it is of prime importance for the health of your body, mind and spirit, in both their internal and their external activities.

The Golden Principles (Chin Tao Li) of T'ai Chi Ch'uan

1. Keep your body erect without stiffness.
2. Everything about you should be completely relaxed, especially the mind.
3. Maintain the heel and toe principles for all foot movements.
4. Co-ordinate the movements of the upper and lower halves of the body.
5. Harmonize the internal and external physical aspects of the body.
6. Ensure that there is a continuity of movement at all times, and that all movements follow a curve or circular form. Movements are never straight lines in T'ai Chi.
7. Study the many Taoist breathing exercises.
8. Learn to breathe deeply through your lower abdomen, and keep your tongue against the roof of your mouth.
9. Extend and let your vitality power flow on all outward movements.
10. Recall and relax your vitality power on all inward movements.
11. Live the Ch'ang Ming way (Taoist macrobiotics).
12. Study the laws of life within the realms of the spiritual path (Tao).
13. Study the use and harmonization of the vitality power and macro-cosmic energy, which are the internal and external, physical and spiritual energies.

Chapter 5

T'ai Chi Stances

There are fourteen basic postures or stances in our T'ai Chi Ch'uan which were laid down originally by the Lee family of very ancient China, and these were named after various animals and birds as was the habit in those far-off days.

Illustrations and descriptions are included in this chapter, and we suggest that before you begin to practise the actual 'form' of T'ai Chi, you learn these various stances and try to move from one to the other smoothly.

Be sure to keep your body upright, without stiffness or tension, so that you remain constantly stable. One good way is to practise in front of a mirror, so that you can constantly watch your posture (body) and your stance (legs) at all times. Remember that you can stand erect without hardness, and you can remain soft without being sloppy. Finding the middle path between the two does not come easily, and it takes a lot of work and practise to acquire it.

Your legs act like the roots of a tree, the body is the trunk, and the arms and hands are the branches and the twigs. Each part is separate, but all have specific jobs to do, so that they work as one — just like the Yin and the Yang and the Tao. You will then find that you can maintain a good and strong balance at all times, and that you will be able to root your feet at any moment.

From the first time you start to practise in any of our classes you will discover that everything you do contains the essence of Chi energy, and you will be taught how to utilize these essences to your maximum power and mental control. Unlike other styles, we teach you how to use and control your Chi energy from the moment you join the class, and help to prove to yourself that Chi is something that you can learn to harness, store and control through your postures, stances and hand movements.

This type of movement is known as 'movement with stillness' (Yun Tung Pu Yun Tung), which is akin to the stillness within the centre of a cyclone, or the tranquillity of the void at the centre of the dynamic forces of the universe. It appears to be insubstantial yet it is enormously substantial. It is the very simple formula of everything, for it is Yin and Yang in complete harmony with one another.

If there is no organized class in your immediate area, remember to practise regularly, especially the following stances, and learn to move from one to another with a heel and toe action, similar to natural walking.

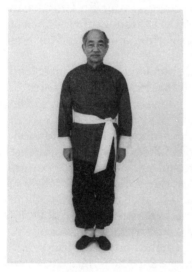

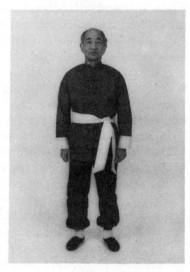

Eagle Stance
(Ying Shih)
Stand with both feet together, heels touching and body upright, eyes looking directly ahead, and arms and hands hanging loosely down by your sides.

Bear Stance
(Hsiung Shih)
Stand with the feet about the width of your shoulders apart, body erect without tension, and arms and hands relaxed by the sides of your thighs.

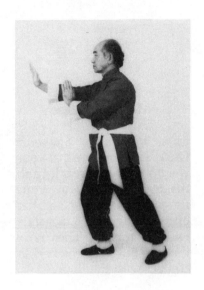

Dragon Stance
(Lung Shih)
From the Eagle or Bear Stance step forward one pace with either your right or left foot, bend the knee, and place 80% of your body weight on to it. Keep your other leg straight, but without tension.

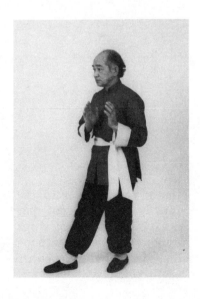

Duck Stance
(Ya Shih)
From the Dragon or Snake Stance slide the front foot back and keep it flat on the floor. Whilst you move your foot back, transfer your body weight on to your rear leg and bend the knee slightly. The front leg should be kept straight.

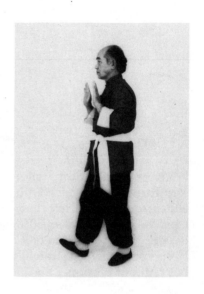

Monkey Stance
(Hou Shih)

From the Dragon, Snake or Duck Stance ensure that your weight is on your rear leg and the knee is bent. Draw your front foot back, keeping it flat on the floor until it can slide back no further. Then raise the toes but keep the heel in contact with the floor.

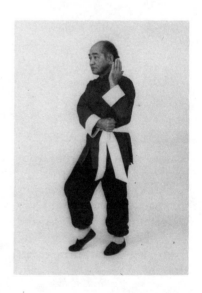

Cat Stance
(Mao Shih)

This is very similar to the Monkey Stance except that once your front foot stops moving raise the heel into the air ensuring that the toes are kept in contact with the floor.

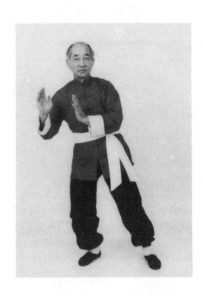

Leopard Stance
(Pao Shih)
From the Bear Stance push one hip out sideways, transfer most of your body weight on to the leg on that side, and bend the knee. The other leg should be kept straight.

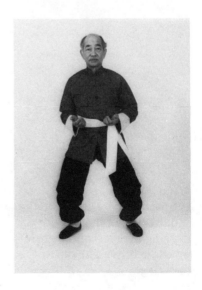

Riding Horse Stance
(Ch'i Ma Shih)
From the Eagle or Bear Stance, step sideways with one foot until both feet are a little more than the width of your shoulders apart. Bend both knees retaining the balance of your body on both legs.

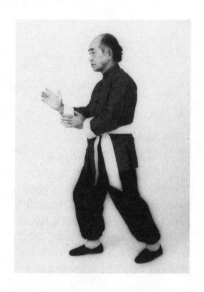

Snake Stance
(She Shih)

From the Eagle or Bear Stance, move one foot about one pace forward, keeping both knees slightly bent and your body weight evenly distributed on both legs.

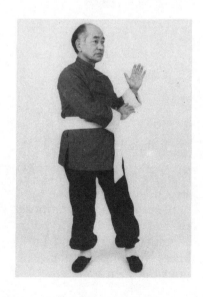

Lion Stance
(Shih Shih)

From the Bear Stance or Leopard Stance, just turn the shoulders to one side (without moving the feet) and transfer your body weight on to the back leg.

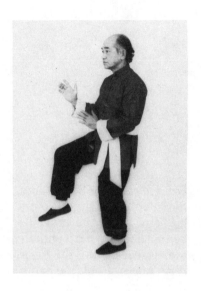

Crane Stance
(Hao Shih)
From the Cat or Monkey Stance, keep your weight on the rear leg, lift your front foot and raise your toes into the air until your thigh is parallel to the floor. When your leg stops moving allow your toes to droop downwards.

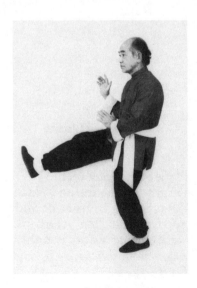

Dog Stance
(Kou Shih)
From the Crane Stance, gently swing your front foot forward and upwards, pulling your toes back (as in the picture). Once the leg stops moving, let your toes drop forward. (The maximum height for a Dog Stance is having the whole leg parallel to the floor).

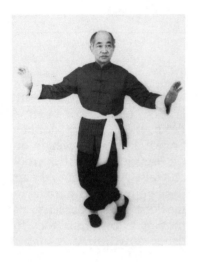

Scissor Stance
(Chien Tao Shih)
From the Eagle or Bear Stance, move your weight on to one leg, and place the other leg behind and beyond it with the toes just touching the floor. Both knees should be bent.

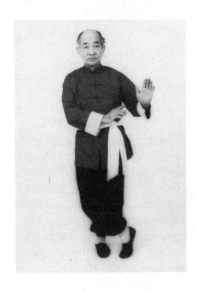

Crossed Leg Stance
(P'anche T'ui Shih)
This is a complete opposition of the Scissor Stance. Put your weight on one leg and place the other leg in front of and across the leg that is supporting your weight. Allow your toes to rest lightly on the floor.

Chapter 6

I Fu Shou
(Adhering or Sticky Hand)

I Fu Shou is a section of T'ai Chi that fascinates every practitioner of the art, and brings to light powers that everyone possesses but very few people realize they have. That is why in some parts of China, I Fu Shou is sometimes called the 'Enlightened Hand'.

I Fu Shou is an exercise in which two people participate. Each person tries to upset the balance of the other whilst maintaining their own stability. Contact is through the arms and hands throughout the exercise. No matter what stance is adopted, there may always be a weakness in the balance of the body whether one moves left or right, backward or forward, upward or downward, and it is by taking advantage of these six directional weaknesses that the participants in I Fu Shou try to 'uproot' each other — to cause the other to lose their footing. The most difficult way to do this is to lift the other off the ground, but even this may be achieved provided that one has practised diligently and developed a faultless technique.

Without a doubt, uprooting your partner by lifting them completely off the ground is the summit of achievement in I Fu Shou, but it is the heightened sensitivity that you develop by being in constant touch with your partner that is the chief value of the exercise. Slowly, and through constant practise, you will be able to tell whether your opponent is at all tense, which of their feet is carrying the most weight, and which part of the foot is experiencing the greatest pressure. You must also estimate the degree of pressure and even the direction in which it is being applied. Thus there is a lot of sensitivity involved, and through your training you will eventually be able to judge your movements so that you can succeed in uprooting your partner.

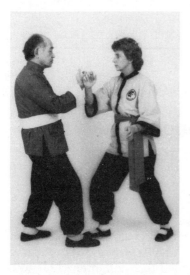 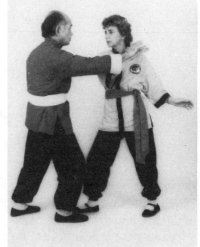

Once you have begun to acquire the sense of being in constant touch, the next step is for you and your partner to close your eyes and practise the same techniques. You will find that this greatly enhances your sensitivity. You will begin to understand what is going on inside your opponent's body, and this will increase your understanding of what is going on inside yourself — your partner becomes a mirror in which you can see your own reflection. If you dedicate yourself to this type of training you will soon find, even if your partner does not move at all the arm or the hand that is in contact with you, that you will be able to tell precisely how and in what direction they are moving the other parts of their body. Ultimately, after a great deal of dedicated practise and expert tuition, you will be able to feel and fully understand the same sensations as your partner, without being in actual physical contact with them at all. This illustrates another important aspect of the ultimate objective of T'ai Chi — hyper-sensitivity.

All aspects of T'ai Chi need dynamic concentration, so that the right and proper technique is used at the right time, and in

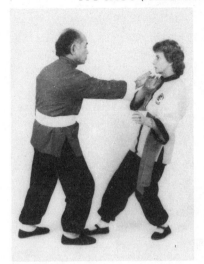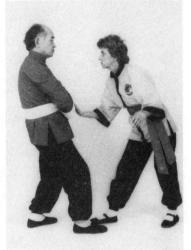

learning this you will acquire greater mind control and a much higher level of mental and emotional consciousness. Through diligent practice you will soon notice a distinctive and marked change in your daily life. You will find that decisions become easier to make, that your reactions become quicker, that you will become more peaceful and relaxed within yourself, and that you gain a much greater control over your emotions. In addition, you will gain complete mastery of your own body and mind, and also develop a superb balance.

To make yourself fully receptive to the tiny muscular changes that take place within the body of your partner, you must first endeavour to relax completely, so that your faculties are at their sharpest. You must also give way to any pressure or force that your opponent may exert against you, no matter how slight or gentle it may be. Your sensitivity must be of such fineness that if a feather were placed on your arm, that arm would slowly sink down because of the weight of it. This is one of the golden rules of I Fu Shou — the power of being tenderly gentle, as delicate as a morning breeze but with the dynamism of a tornado and the force of a hurricane.

It now remains to describe some of the simple basic movements, and to outline the various stages so that you can find the path to the complete mastery of I Fu Shou.

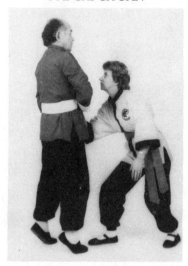

To begin with you will need a partner to train with, and to share the delicate situations that will arise when you start learning to feel and interpret the changes in touch. The two of you should stand facing one another, each with your right foot placed forward of your left foot and your body weight evenly distributed on both legs. This is the Snake Stance (She Shih), which is a completely neutral stance. Your right foot should be placed alongside your partner's right foot but not touching it; both of you should have your knees slightly bent and the body upright but without stiffness. Having adopted this posture, raise your right arm (your partner does the same) and hold it against your partner's, with the wrists lightly touching. This is the type of contact that must be maintained throughout your training session, although the actual point of contact will vary as you commence your movements.

As we have mentioned before, there are six points of weakness in every stance. These weaknesses can be very noticeable irrespective of the stance or posture that your partner may adopt during your progression in the arts. These weaknesses are (1) to the right, (2) to the left, (3) directly forward, (4) directly backward, (5) downwards, and (6) upwards. Both of you should endeavour to find these weaknesses, and having found them through touch, try to take advantage of them to upset each other's balance. In time, with more experience and advanced techniques, you will be able to uproot each other completely in all six directions.

Now let us assume that your opponent gently pushes forward towards your chest. Directly you feel the pressure, give way by slowly transferring your body weight on to your left leg, thereby moving your body weight backwards; as you do so turn your shoulders to your right. You will immediately notice that your partner is now pushing nothing, just the air, and in so doing is becoming more unstable in their balance. If you now gently extend your arm, you will find that you can topple them to their left.

Again let your partner push directly towards your chest, and now give way by transferring your weight on to your rear leg and turning to the right, but this time make a big circle with your right hand, first out to your right then inwards towards your partner so that their arm touches their chest or shoulders. You will find that you can now gently topple them to their right (your left).

You must keep your feet firmly planted on the floor at all times, so that you maintain a good balance and stability at all times. If you move one of your feet even the slightest to retain your balance, then you have been uprooted and your partner has won.

While you must keep in contact with your partner at all times, you can shift the point of contact to your hand or to a different part of your arm for instance by rotating your arm or hand around your opponent's. Provided that you do not lose touch, you can move your arm and hand in any direction — forward, backward, upward, downward, to the side — always with a view to exploiting your partner's weaknesses and uprooting them. Experiment a little and try every conceivable angle of contact, and when you have done this using your right arm, practise the same techniques using your left arm and hand and with your left foot forward (your partner doing the same).

Once you have fully mastered the techniques of using one arm and hand, the next stage is to bring both arms and hands into play. You will find that there are now enormous possibilities opening up for you, but there are also a number of golden rules which have to be adhered to and borne in mind. If you want to change hands at any time, make sure that one hand is always in contact with your partner. If you have both hands touching them at the same time, be sure not to let your energy flow out of them at the same time; this is called 'double weighting' (Shuang Chung), and it restricts the amount of energy that can be concentrated on any one object. It is better to let your vitality flow out of one hand or arm, while resting the other lightly on your partner. Similarly, you can shift your weight from one leg to the other, but do not allow your weight to rest on both legs at the same time. This is also double weighting; it could leave you exposed, and therefore much easier to uproot.

The next stage is to practise the same techniques from different stances. This is a difficult stage to master because you have to think simultaneously of your arm and hand movements, the advancement or retirement of your legs, the angles of your body, and the constant change of your weight distribution. To start with it is best to change the basic stance only by moving one of your feet forward or back a pace. Gradually you will find that you can incorporate more and more difficult stances and still achieve the same mastery.

The final stage, which can only be mastered with the help of expert tuition, is to learn how to uproot your partner completely by affecting their state of balance in such a way that you can lift them completely off the floor with your arm and hand techniques. To achieve this very advanced form of uprooting requires complete dedication over many years of practise, but it is within the realms of possibility for everyone.

Anyone can throw a stone into a pool of water and cause a splash and many ripples, but your ultimate aim should be to throw your pebble into the same pool without causing even the slightest splash, even a single ripple. You can succeed given time, practise, dedication and strong mental control, so set your mind on the ultimate goal.

Chapter 7

Whirling Arms and Hands

Like I Fu Shou, Whirling Arms (Lun Pei) and Whirling Hands (Lun Shou) encourage the development of quick mental and physical reactions and a high level of sensitivity. Both are characterized, as their names suggest, by circular movements of the arms and hands. They are competitive in spirit but completely without violence, and indirectly they teach simple basic principles of self-defence.

The two arts include techniques to ward off, parry and deflect thrusts that may be made towards your body, and with constant practise you can develop the ability to recognize your partner's intentions before they are carried out. You will learn how to feel and exploit the weaknesses in their movements and postures, and in so doing you will come to understand your own weaknesses and develop greater concentration and awareness. You will build the foundations for a stronger balance, learn how to effectively synchronize your body movements, and become much more sensitive and perceptive. In addition to all these, the control and utilization of your Chi energy plays a very big part in your practise.

Whirling Arms (Lun Pei)
To begin with take up the Snake Stance (right foot forward alongside your partner's right foot; knees slightly bent for greater flexibility), and raise your right arm so that the back of your wrist is just touching the back of your partner's right wrist (your partner

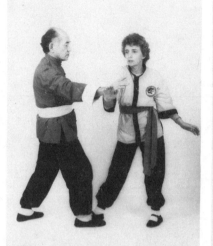
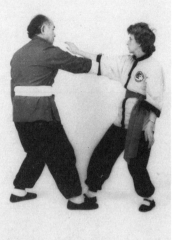

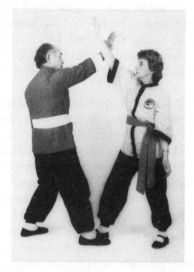

of course, should take up the same posture). Next start to circle your arm to your right, and as you do so, your partner should allow their own right arm to rotate freely, thereby giving way to the slightest pressure from you. As your arm circles, you should endeavour to alter the size of the circle, making small, medium-size, large and extra large rotations.

After a little while, your partner may decide to take the initiative and rotate their arm the other way. As soon as you feel the opposing pressure, immediately give way. So the exercise continues, each giving way to the other when necessary, yet each trying to take command as the situation changes. The object is to touch your partner's head, chest or stomach with the hand of the rotating arm, but you should not straighten your arm to make the touch, which should be very gentle, and you must endeavour to make the touch while you continue to rotate your arm. In addition to the arm movement, you may also move your body backwards or forwards, or turn your shoulders and hips, but any movement at the top must not effect the bottom, and you should keep your feet absolutely stationary. Moving the body not only keeps it very supple but it makes it easier for you to evade the touches, and so makes it much more difficult for your partner to get through your defence system.

The next stage of Whirling Arms is to learn how to use the rotations of your arm so as to rock your partner's balance. When your technique is good enough, you will be able to uproot them completely, but to achieve this requires a great deal of practice.

Once you have mastered the technique of using one arm, the next step is to use both arms, either simultaneously or alternatively, but you should ensure that when changing from one to the other you do not lose contact with your partner's arm. You may circle your arms in opposite directions from each other, or both arms can rotate in the same direction. You may also vary the area of circulation by rotating one arm in a large circle whilst the other one makes small circlets. The variety of possible movements is enormous, and to achieve mastery of the techniques for using both arms requires considerable experience, extremely rapid reactions, a high level of body control, and great mental agility and concentration.

Finally, there is the further art of moving your feet according to specified patterns, at the same time making full use of your body. To reach this stage usually takes about three years of constant training, and to conquer it is extremely difficult. Sheer dedication together with expert tuition is required to gain the full appreciation and understanding of the art.

Whirling Hands (Lun Shou)

While there is a superficial similarity between Whirling Hands and Whirling Arms, the two are very different from each other as regards approach, technique, and feel. The object is to touch your opponent's body or head with either your fingertips or elbow (which sounds quite easy until you start to practise) and, at a later stage, to upset your partner's balance and uproot them.

The initial stance that you and your partner must adopt is the same as in Whirling Arms, but this time you must interlock your fingers with your partner — your right hand with their left, and their right with your left. Next, keeping your elbows bent at all times, begin to rotate your hands, either both together or each one separately, in large, medium or small circles. How you are able to rotate them will depend, of course, on your partner's reactions and manoeuvres. By turning your body, twisting your shoulders, bending forward or backward, turning your wrists and shifting your balance, you should, once you have acquired skill and perfection, be able to touch your partner without being touched yourself. If your legs begin to ache, then with mutual consent with your partner you can both change your stance, so that your left feet are forward and your right behind.

When you have mastered the initial stage of Whirling Hands, you can progress to the later stages, which involve learning how

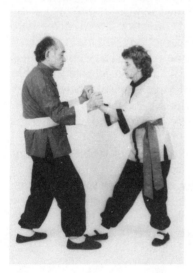
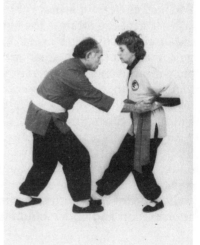

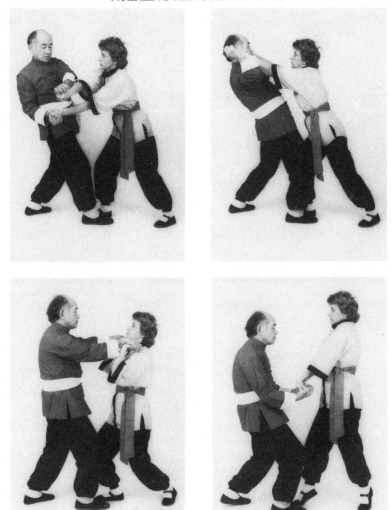

to uproot your partner and move your feet.

From the point of view of self-defence, both Whirling Arms and Whirling Hands are excellent training, and teach you hand-to-hand techniques at close quarters. Once you have learned the basic stages, you will thoroughly enjoy participating in the battle of wits and practising the skills that are involved.

Chapter 8

T'ai Chi Sword (T'ai Chi Chien)

T'ai Chi Sword makes full use of the combined techniques of Whirling Hands and Whirling Arms, but these are made more difficult by the weight and length of the sword. Greater mental concentration is required to retain complete control of the arms, wrists and hands, while maintaining perfect balance, especially in a few sequences where the whole body makes a complete whirl to demonstrate the 'order of the universe'. These techniques are not easy, but nothing is really easy in the full art of T'ai Chi, because there is so much to remember and so many movements have to be practised in order to understand the essence of energy and force, and expand self-awareness and mental control.

In accordance with the basic principles of T'ai Chi, the 'Sword' form, which comprises 216 movements, has no straight lines. Movements are performed in circular motion, with excellent balance and perfect utilization of the body in the movement from one stance to another in a gentle and continuous flow. These movements enrich bodily health, and can eventually eliminate all stress and strain. Whilst outwardly there is a great physical activity, inwardly there is peace and tranquility, a perfect balance of Yin and Yang. This balance enables us to become one with ourselves, and such an integral part of our everyday life, that this harmony can also protect us like a shield.

It is not possible to include the whole 'form' of T'ai Chi Sword in this introduction. I hope to describe it in detail in a future volume, but the following photographs may give you an impression of the beautiful flow of movements that are involved in T'ai Chi Sword.

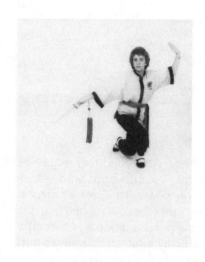

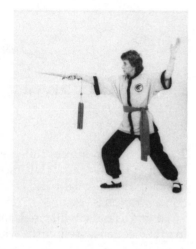

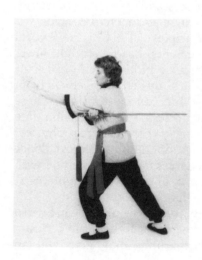

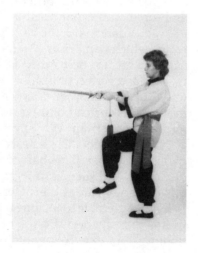

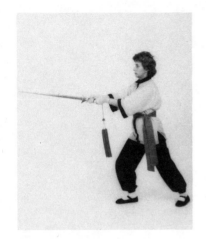

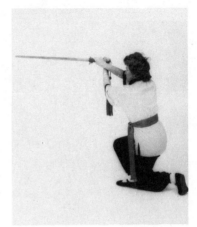

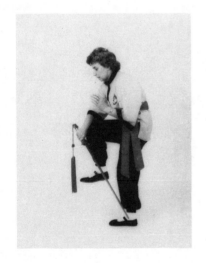

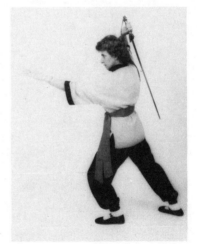

Chapter 9

T'ai Chi Dance

T'ai Chi Dance is not a dance as most Westerners would imagine it. It is not normally performed to music but it can be. Unlike T'ai Chi Sword which is based on the 'order of the universe' and the phenomena within it, T'ai Chi Dance has its foundations in the Five Elements and Li energy, the general directions of the flow of these, and their respective colours.

Foot, leg and body movements, balance and graceful flow take first priority in T'ai Chi Dance. Concentration on the complete harmony of movement is absolutely essential if the subtlety of the postures and stances are to be achieved correctly.

T'ai Chi Dance is a beautiful tapestry of motion, gentle in its flow, graceful in its execution, and creating an air of complete tranquillity. Motion and stillness are a wonderful balance to each other. There is also a complete 'form' of T'ai Chi Dance, but it is the baby of all the 'forms' that we do, for it is only about 400 years old. You will gain some impression of its gracefulness from the few photographs included here.

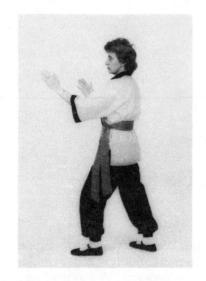

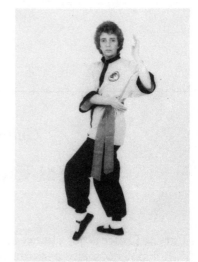

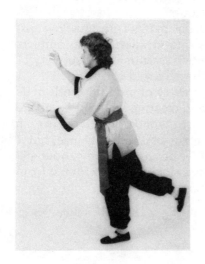

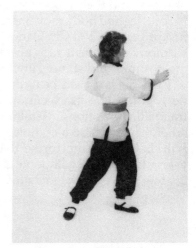

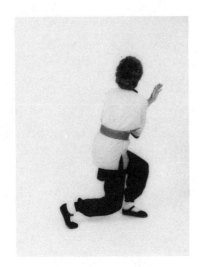

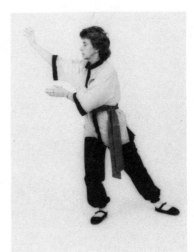

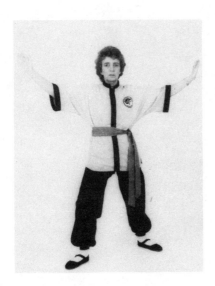

Chapter 10

T'ai Chi Stick

Like all the other sections of T'ai Chi, T'ai Chi Stick is an integral part of a complete art. It can only be mastered after long and dedicated practise with expert guidance, for it too contains many deep essences.

Some idea may be gained from the following illustrations, but its true beauty and value cannot be appreciated until you have witnessed it yourself, or better still, begun to master the movements, techniques and essences for yourself.

Very few schools teach T'ai Chi Sword, T'ai Chi Dance and T'ai Chi Stick, but all of these are taught within our Taoist Arts, for they represent our links with Taoist antiquity, and keep us in touch with our ancient Masters.

Taken together, all of the Taoist arts are like a hand. Take any one of them away, and it is like a hand with no fingers. Each is separate in its own right yet all are one, for they combine, blend and harmonize together, not only through technique, stances, postures and movement, but also because they help to reinforce each other with the control, use and flow of the essences that are involved.

The following photographs of T'ai Chi Stick will help to convey an impression of the art. One day we hope to produce a book that will give you all 270 movements, for we feel sure that you will love the depths that it contains within itself, and the elation that it can create.

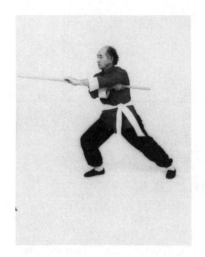
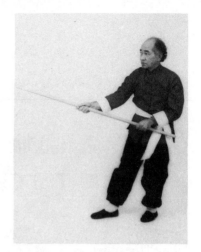

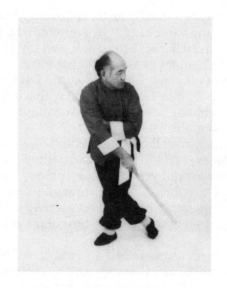

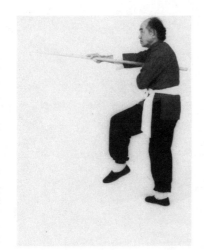
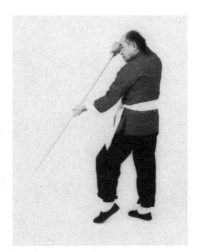

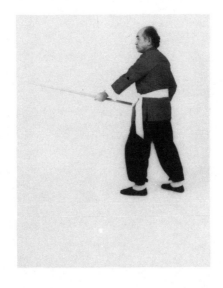

Chapter 11

The Sequences of T'ai Chi Ch'uan

The original eight postures, which came into being some 10,000 years ago, were increased to a total of thirteen when the very first T'ai Chi sequences were formulated. This book still retains the original animal names of each stance, which were first adopted by the ancient Taoists of China, and by the Lee family.

However, when T'ai Chi became more widely known within China, many schools and classes were founded, and their teachers tried to hide the techniques, stances, sequences and sets behind a facade of words, such as 'The Crane Spreads its Wings', 'Hit the Tiger', and 'Brush Knee and Side Step', which enabled them to retain some originality for themselves.

For the benefit of all our readers, including those who are truly interested in and dedicated to every aspect of our Chinese Taoist Arts, we are specifying the ancient animal name of each stance. Here is the more modern description of each sequence of movements, but it is interesting to be aware that even these were devised some 1,500 years ago.

1-3	Gather Celestial Energy
4-6	Play the Guitar
7-11	Fair Lady Weaving
12-17	The Crane Exercises its Wings
18-20	Drive the Tiger Away
21-22	Grasp the Bird's Tail
23-24	Brush Knee and Side Step

Chapter 12

The Form of T'ai Chi Ch'uan

Preparation

Eagle Stance
(Ying Shih)
Stand with your front facing towards the South and your back towards the North. East should then be to your left and West to your right. Now stand with your feet together with both heels in contact with one another, but the toes pointing slightly outward. Let your arms hang down so that your open hands lay loosely by the sides of your thighs. The body should be erect but completely relaxed, and your eyes should be looking directly ahead. The mind should be tranquil and you should feel at peace with yourself.

Bear Stance
(Hsiung Shih)
Step directly to your left with your left foot, ensuring that you execute a heel and toe action with that foot, until both feet are about a shoulder-width apart. Your arms and hands should remain as before, hanging loosely by your thighs. Whilst your body and head have remained in the same position, ensure that your body weight is evenly distributed on both legs.
(See page 71 for photographs of this sequence).

Preparation: left — Eagle Stance; right — Bear Stance.

Sequence 1: Gather Celestial Energy

1. Eagle Stance
(Ying Shih)

Slowly raise your hands and create a half circling movement round your hips. Bring your hands together in front of your lower abdomen about two inches below the navel. The tips of the fingers of both hands should point to each other, but should not actually touch. The palms of the hands should be facing down to the floor. Your elbows will naturally move outwards as you execute the above movement. Simultaneously draw your left foot in until it is alongside your right foot.

2. Eagle Stance
(Ying Shih)

Now slowly raise both arms and hands to a point directly above your head by taking them forward and upward in an arc, until the palms of the hands face towards the ceiling or sky. About halfway through this movement, your hands will be on a level with your eyes — at this point let your eyes follow the back of your hands until the maximum vertical point is reached. This will mean that you will have to tilt your head back during the execution of this movement, but there should be no strain or stress. Ensure that the fingertips of both hands still point to each other.

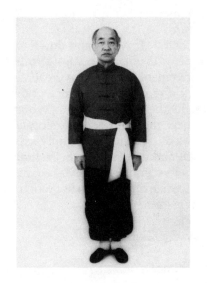

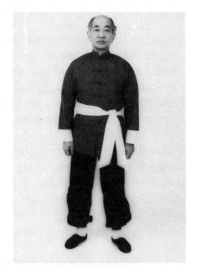

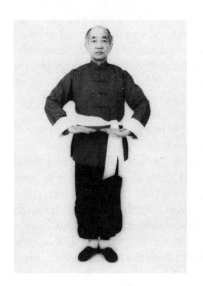

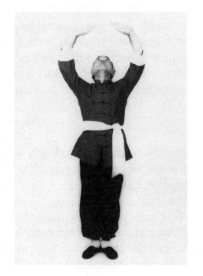

1   2

3. Eagle Stance
(Ying Shih)

Lower both of your hands in a half circle forward and down to a point in front of the lower abdomen. As you do so, allow your head and eyes to follow this movement, until your head is naturally erect and your eyes look directly ahead. Once your hands reach your lower abdomen, let the tension go out of your hands so the fingers point downwards, then immediately slowly rotate both wrists so that the palms of the hands face upward. You will notice that both hands will make a small circle, so that they arrive at a point two inches below your navel. Make sure that the fingers of both hands point to each other but do not touch, and keep them straight without tension.

Sequence 2: Play the Guitar

4. Dragon Stance
(Lung Shih)

Step directly forward one pace with your right foot, and once the foot comes in contact with the floor place 80% of your body weight on to it. Bend your right knee, but keep your left leg straight. At the same time as you step, move your hands forward and outward in an arc, rotating on your elbows, and keep the palms of both hands uppermost, with the fingers pointing directly forward. The right hand should be one hand's length ahead of your left hand, and both arms roughly parallel to the floor.

5. Monkey Stance
(Hou Shih)

Slowly transfer your body weight on to your left leg and bend the left knee slightly, and as you do this allow your right foot to slide back towards you. Once your foot stops moving, raise the right toes, ensuring that you keep your heel in contact with the floor. As you transfer your body weight, turn your hands outward and then upward by rotating your wrists. These two half circles should be about the size of a football, and the left hand is kept behind the right hand. Now draw both hands back towards your navel by bending your elbows more deeply.

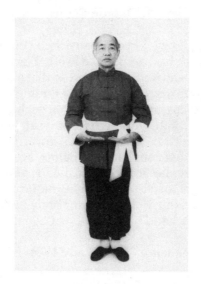

3

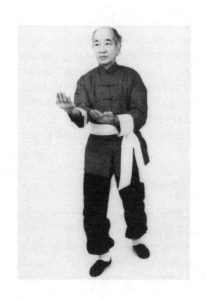

4

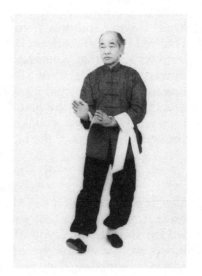

5

6. Dragon Stance
(Lung Shih)

Pivot on your left leg whilst you slowly circle your right foot ninety degrees to your right, so you face West. Place your right foot on the floor and bend your right knee so that about 80% of your body weight is transferred to it. Adjust the angle of your left foot with a heel and toe movement, and straighten your left leg. Simultaneously rotate your wrists so that your hands hang downwards, then circle them inwards towards your body, and finally turn them over so that both palms face upward. Having completed the circular action of the hands allow both arms to swing to your right to follow the turning movement of your body. Keep your elbows fairly close to your body, and your left hand behind your right hand.

Sequence 3: Fair Lady Weaving

7. Monkey Stance
(Hou Shih)

Transfer your body weight slowly onto your left leg and at the same time draw your right foot back and slightly bend your left knee. Having withdrawn your foot about twelve inches, raise your right toes off the floor. Whilst moving into this stance, rotate both wrists so that your hands make a half circle, outward and upward, about the size of a football. Then draw both arms back towards your sides, making sure that both palms face each other and that your arms are parallel. Now bend your body slightly forward, keeping your back straight, so that you can look down between the palms of the hands.

8. Dragon Stance
(Lung Shih)

Move your right foot forward and transfer the weight of the body on to it, making sure that your right knee is bent and that your left leg straightens. As you effect the leg movements, rotate your wrists so that at first your hands droop, then circle inwards towards your body, then move upwards so that the palms of your hands arrive directly in front of the shoulders. Now slowly straighten both arms by pushing forward with the back of your hands.

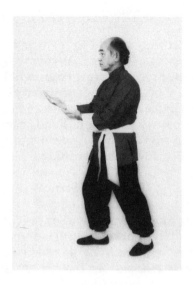

6

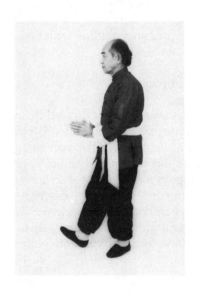

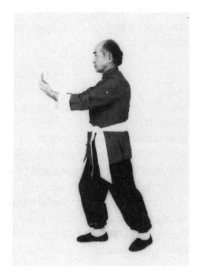

7 8

9. Monkey Stance
(Hou Shih)

Slowly move your body weight to the rear and onto your left leg with your left knee slightly bent. As your weight is withdrawn, with the same slow precision draw your right foot back until it rests on the heel a short distance away from your left foot, then slowly raise your right toes into the air. Simultaneously, bend your elbows and slowly bring your hands back until they stop a short distance in front of their respective shoulders, with the fingers still pointing towards the ceiling.

10. Dragon Stance
(Lung Shih)

Move your right foot forward, and once it rests on the floor transfer your body weight on to it, bend your right knee and straighten your left leg. The body should be kept erect without stiffness, and the eyes should look directly ahead. Whilst moving your right foot, rotate your wrists, so that your hands circle forward, outward, then back in front of the shoulders — at the end of the movement the palms of both hands should face directly forward. Now gently and slowly push both hands forward and straighten both arms, keeping them on a straight line with your shoulders.

11. Monkey Stance
(Hou Shih)

Slowly withdraw your body until your weight is fully resting on your left leg, but keep the left knee slightly bent. With the withdrawal of your weight bring your right foot back by allowing it to slide along the floor until it is a short distance ahead of your left foot. Once your right foot stops moving, raise the toes of your right foot, but keep the heel in contact with the floor. As you commence your weight transfer, bend both elbows and slowly draw your hands back, still on a line with the shoulders, letting them stop a short distance away from your body with both palms facing outward.

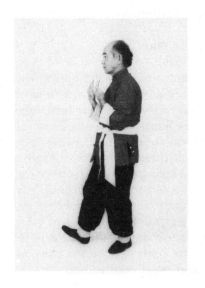

9

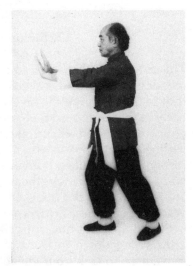

10

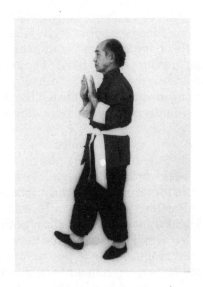

11

Sequence 4: The Crane Exercises its Wings

12. Riding Horse Stance
(Ch'i Ma Shih)

This can be a little tricky, so concentrate. First of all lower the toes of your right foot, but before they touch the floor, turn your foot to the left, pivoting on the heel. As you do this, turn your body to the left too, so that you face South once more. Now lift your left toes, and while you pivot on your left heel, swing your left toes slightly to the left and lower them to the floor. As you turn your body allow both arms to swing down in front of the body, then slowly move them outwards and upwards until they are parallel with the floor, on a level with your shoulders. As you complete these arm movements, point the fingers of your left hand upwards and your right hand fingers down. As your arms swing down in front of your body, allow the flow of movement to sink your weight and bend your knees.

13. Leopard Stance
(Pao Shih)

Lean to your right, transferring your body weight on to your right leg, and at the same time bend your right knee and straighten your left leg. As this happens allow your arms to swing down towards the floor, then upwards in front of your abdomen. Now let your right hand rise so that it stops in front of your left shoulder with the palm facing inward, whilst the left hand is slightly bent to form a cup just underneath your right elbow.

14. Eagle Stance
(Ying Shih)

Draw your left foot inwards towards your right foot until both heels touch and your toes are turned slightly outwards. Once your feet are together, straighten your body and distribute your weight evenly on both legs. Whilst doing this, allow both arms to swing downwards. The left arm should be moved to your left side, with your left open hand nestling close to your left thigh. Your right arm should continue its motion in a big circular arc, outwards and upwards, until your right hand is above and in front of your head. Your right palm should face directly forward, and your right fingers should be pointing to your left (or Eastwards).

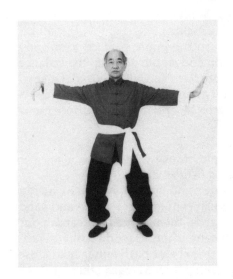

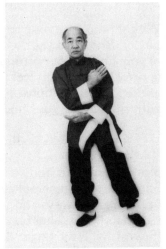

12

13

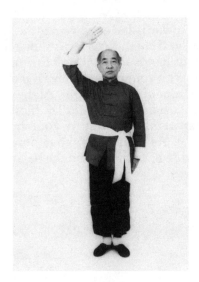

14

15. Eagle Stance
(Ying Shih)

Without moving your feet, turn the upper part of your body ninety degrees to your left and endeavour to keep the balance of your body in the centre of both feet. You will need strict mental control to keep both feet firmly rooted to the floor. Both arms are kept in the positions of Stance 14, and they should both move with the turn of your body.

16. Eagle Stance
(Ying Shih)

Slowly turn your body to your right, so that you face directly South once again. Simultaneously, circle your left arm and hand outwards, sideways and upwards, then inwards towards your right hand. The palms of both hands should face directly forward (South), with the fingers and thumbs of both hands held close together, and the fingertips pointing towards each other and held a few inches apart.

17. Riding Horse Stance
(Ch'i Ma Shih)

Circle both arms outwards and downwards, then upwards in front of your abdomen and chest. Both arms should cross in front of the chest, and your hands should finish their movement by the sides of your jaws with your palms facing your cheeks. Your right arm should be in front of your left arm. At the same time slowly move your left foot sideways to your left (East), until both feet are a little wider apart than the width of your shoulders, and bend both knees deeply. As your arms move downwards let your weight also sink down, but maintain the balance of your body evenly on both legs.

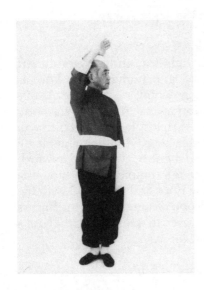

15

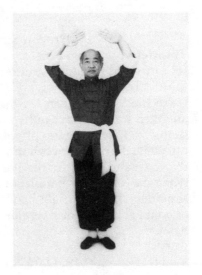
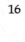

16

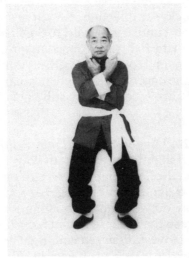

17

Sequence 5: Drive the Tiger Away

18. Dragon Stance *(Lung Shih)*

Transfer your weight on to your right leg, and move your left foot forward (South) about one pace, bending the left knee as the foot rests on the floor, and straightening the right leg. As this is executed, let both arms swing downward in front of the body and then start to move outward. At this point, the left arm will swing back over the top of your left knee with the palm facing up, while the right arm continues to swing outward and upward, then over and inward until it has made a complete circle, stopping when the forearm is parallel to the floor and on a level with the shoulders. Let your right hand droop down, and lift the fingers of your left hand. You have now started to wrestle with the tiger's head.

19. Duck Stance *(Ya Shih)*

With your left foot step back one pace behind your right foot, and as soon as it rests on the floor, bend your left knee and place most of your body weight on to it. Your right foot should remain flat on the floor. As you move your left leg, rotate both arms in circles in a clockwise direction, the left arm going outward, upward and inward until it is parallel to the floor on a level with the shoulders, and the right arm going outward, downward and inward until the palm faces upwards. Let your left hand droop down, and raise the fingers of your right hand. Imagine encircling a big ball in both arms, for you are still having problems with the tiger's head.

20. Dragon Stance *(Lung Shih)*

Step forward and slightly outward with your right foot, and as soon as it rests on the floor, put your weight on to it, bend your right knee, and straighten your left leg. Let your left hand swing down and slightly outward until it is alongside your left thigh, lifting the fingers so that your left palm faces the floor. As your left arm starts to move, you sweep your right arm down in front of your body, then forward and upward in an arc until it reaches shoulder level. The fingers of your right should be tipped slightly to the left, and the right palm should face directly forward.

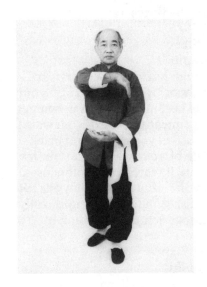

18

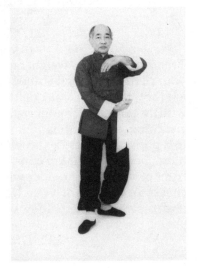

19

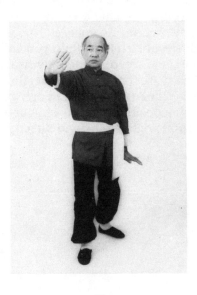

20

Sequence 6: Grasp the Bird's Tail

21. Cat Stance
(Mao Shih)

Transfer your body weight on to your left leg, slowly draw back
your right foot until it is about eight or twelve inches from your
left foot, then raise your right heel keeping your toes in contact
with the floor. Move your right arm inwards towards your waist,
clenching your right hand into a fist as you do so, and bring it
to a position alongside the left side of your waist. Lift your left
hand, bending your left elbow, until it reaches a position just in
front of your left shoulder with your left palm facing your left
cheek. At this point your right fist should be fitting directly
underneath your left elbow, without actually touching it.

22. Dragon Stance
(Lung Shih)

Turn ninety degrees to your right (West), circling your right foot
with the turn of your body. Now step one pace forward,
transferring your weight on to your right leg, and bend the right
knee. As soon as your weight has been adjusted, correct the angle
of your left foot by pivoting on your left heel as you move your
toes, then straighten your left leg. Whilst you are turning, let your
arms move in the same arc, but gradually straighten your right
arm and lift it slightly, so that it arrives over the top of your right
leg at shoulder level. Following the same arc, your left hand will
slowly move from a position in front of your left shoulder to a
point just inside your right elbow and directly in front of your
right breast.

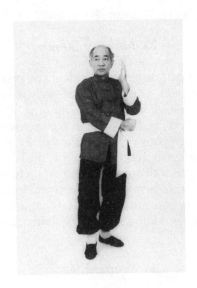

21

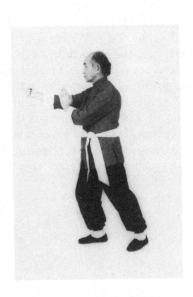

22

Sequence 7: Brush Knee and Side Step

23. Monkey Stance
(Hou Shih)

Transfer your weight on to your left leg, and bend your left knee whilst you draw back your right foot. When you cannot draw it back any further and the foot stops moving, lift your right toes but ensure that your right heel is in contact with the floor. At the same time, open your right hand and make an inverted figure 's' movement with your hand, starting at the bottom. When you get to the top of the 's' drop your hand down towards your right knee. You will have to bend slightly forward, but try to keep your back as straight as you can, without any strain or tension. Your left hand, whilst remaining stationary, will dip slightly with the bend of your body.

24. Leopard Stance
(Pao Shih)

Start to transfer your weight, very slowly, on to your right leg, and as you do so, slowly turn your body ninety degrees to your left (South). Your right foot, pivoting on its heel, should naturally follow the turn of your body. When your body has stopped moving drop your right toes down on to the floor, and adjust the angle of your left foot with a heel and toe movement. At this point all your weight should be on your right leg. Rotate both hands in front of the body, with the right hand making the bigger circle. The rotation should be downwards then upwards, until both hands reach a point above and beyond your right shoulder. The palms of both hands should face upwards, and the fingers should be pointing to the right (West). Now turn your head so that it looks to the left (East).

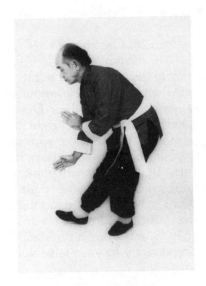

23

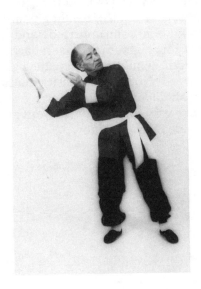

24

Sequence 8: Repulse the Monkey

25. Cat Stance
(Mao Shih)

Turn your body ninety degrees to your left (East), pulling back your left foot, and when the foot stops moving raise your heel but keep your toes in contact with the floor. During this movement you will have to adjust the angle of your right foot by lifting your right toes and pivoting on the heel. Let your arms swing in the same direction as your body and keep both hands open. Now bend your left arm so that your fingers point upwards towards the ceiling, and your left thumb is close to the front of your left shoulder. Swing your right arm round in a big arc with the turn of the body, so that your right forearm is on a level with your waist, and your right thumb is under your left elbow, with your left fingers pointing directly to your left (North).

26. Dragon Stance
(Lung Shih)

Step forward one pace with your left foot, and transfer 80% of your weight on to your left leg, bending your left knee. At the same time turn your right palm uppermost and gently swing your right hand out to your right, then circle it back to a position just in front of your right shoulder, turning the palm of the hand so that it faces forward. Now gently push your hand forward on a line with your shoulder, until your arm is straight. Your left hand should move very slowly from in front of the left shoulder to a position inside the right elbow.

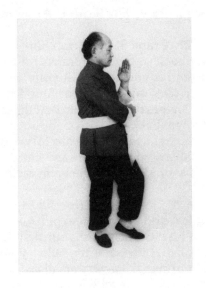

25

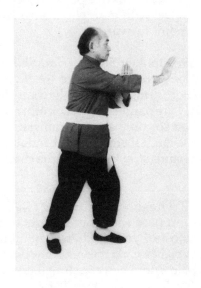

26

Sequence 9: The Stork is Aroused

27. Crane Stance *(Hao Shih)*

Move your body back so that you transfer all your weight on to your right leg, and as you do so raise your left leg into the air, keeping your left toes raised. When your leg stops moving upward, let your left toes dip downward. At the same time swing your right arm down, back, and up on the outside of your right shoulder, with your right palm still facing forward. The left hand makes a very small arc, downwards and back to a position in front of the right shoulder, with the palm facing down.

28. Dog Stance *(Kou Shih)*

Extend your left leg, and as you do so pull your left toes back. Raise the leg to at least the height of your right knee, then drop your left toes forward. At the same time allow your arms to open, and let your right arm make a very small arc downwards then out to your right until it is level with your shoulders, with the fingers pointing to the right. Your left arm will make a bigger arc downwards and forwards to a position just outside your left leg, but still on a level with your shoulders. The fingers of the left hand should point forward.

29. Monkey Stance *(Hou Shih)*

Lower your left foot straight down to the floor, then raise the toes. Now bring both arms inward to the centre line of the body, and as soon as they are parallel with each other, droop the hands and rotate the wrists so your palms face upward. Now move both hands outward and circle them inward, bending the elbow a little more, until both hands stop in front of the chest with the palms facing forward.

30. Dragon Stance *(Lung Shih)*

Step forward a short pace with your left foot, bending your left knee, and place most of your body weight on to your left leg, straightening your right leg. At the same time push gently forward with your open palms until you can straighten your arms, which should be on a level with your shoulders.

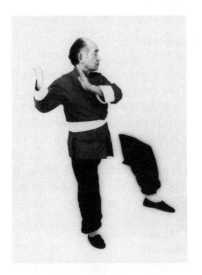

27

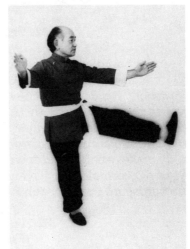

28

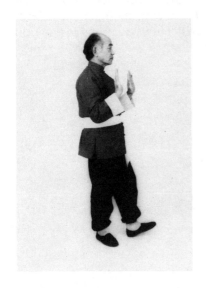

29

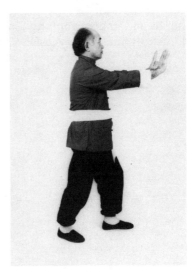

30

Sequence 10: The Double Whip

31. Snake Stance
(She Shih)

Transfer part of your body weight on to your right leg, and draw your left foot back slightly. When the movement is completed, your body weight should be evenly distributed on both legs. Move your arms downwards, then upwards, in a wide circular action, bringing the right arm fully stretched above your right shoulder, with the fingers pointing straight up to the ceiling. The left hand only makes a half circle, downwards and then upwards towards your right armpit, and, having arrived there, the left fingers point upwards and the left palm faces outward (South).

32. Leopard Stance
(Pao Shih)

Turn your body ninety degrees to your right (South) and move your left foot about six inches to your left, placing the majority of your weight on to it. At the same time bend your left knee and adjust your right foot. Circle both arms downwards and then outwards, until they are on a level with your shoulders, with both hands and fingers pointing upwards. Turn your head so that you look to your right (West).

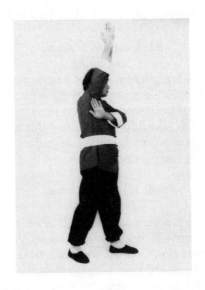

31

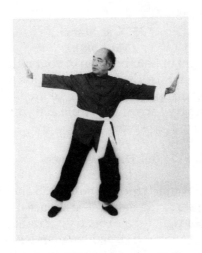

32

Sequence 11: The Cobra Unwinds

33. Leopard Stance
(Pao Shih)
Slowly transfer the weight of your body from your left leg to your right leg, and as you do so move both arms downward then upwards in front of your body, so that your right hand finishes in front of your left shoulder, with the palm inward. Your left hand should stop by your waistline just under your right elbow, with the left palm facing downwards.

34. Dragon Stance
(Lung Shih)
Step forward a pace with your left foot, bending your left knee, putting the majority of your weight on to your left leg, and straightening your right leg. At the same time, swing your left arm forward and upward level with your shoulder, with the palm facing outward. Meanwhile, drop your right hand alongside your right thigh, with the palm facing down and the fingers pointing to your right.

35. Cat Stance
(Mao Shih)
Transfer the weight of your body on to your right leg. Draw your left foot back, then raise the heel, keeping the toes on the floor. Then circle your arms in towards the centre line of your body, with your left arm bent across your front and your right arm fitting behind it forming a 'T' shape.

36. Dragon Stance
(Lung Shih)
Bring the heel of your left foot to the ground and circle your right foot ninety degrees to the right (West). Place most of your body weight on to your right leg and bend your right knee. Adjust the angle of your left foot and straighten your left leg. Rotate your right wrist so that the palm faces upwards, and move your right arm so that it follows the arc of your right leg. Your left arm should follow in the wake of your right arm, and your left hand should stop just inside your right elbow.

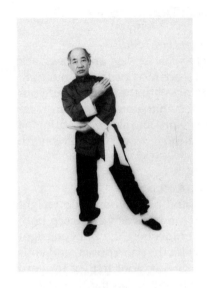

33

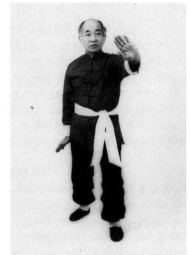

34

35

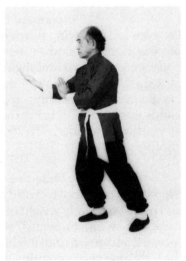

36

Sequence 12: The Wild Dog Retaliates

37. Monkey Stance *(Hou Shih)*
Withdraw your body weight on to your left leg, and draw back
your right leg. When the right foot stops moving, raise your right
toes but keep the right heel in contact with the floor. Bend your
left knee. Rotate your left wrist so that your left palm faces
upward, and sweep both hands outward and sideways, bringing
them both round in an arc to a position in front of the chest with
both palms facing forward.

38. Dog Stance *(Kou Shih)*
Lower the toes of your right foot and place your body weight
on to your right leg. Straighten your arms as you sweep both
hands away from your body, at shoulder height, until your right
hand points directly to your right with the palm down, and your
left hand points directly forward. Swing your left leg forward
and upwards, ensuring that you keep your leg straight, until your
left foot touches the palm or fingers of your left hand. (If you
cannot lift your leg that high, don't worry — do the best you can.)

39. Leopard Stance *(Pao Shih)*
Let your left leg swing down to a position diagonally to the left
of your right leg, and as soon as it touches the floor put your
body weight on to it and slightly bend your left knee. Your right
foot should remain flat on the floor, but straighten your right
leg. Swing both arms upward and to your left, clenching both
hands into fists, and bring them to a point just above the level
of your left shoulder. The insides of your fists should face one
another.

40. Dragon Stance *(Lung Shih)*
Move your right foot forward a few inches, bend your right knee,
and place your body weight on to your right leg. Open your right
hand and swing it upward, above the level of your head, then
forward and down until it is in front of your right shoulder, with
the little finger edge pointing towards the floor. At the same time
your left fist should arc forward and down to a position in front
of your solar plexus, with your left elbow still bent.

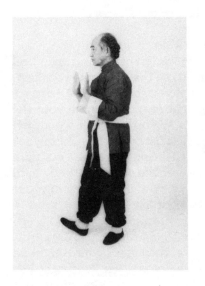

37

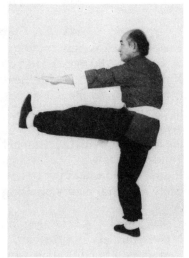

38

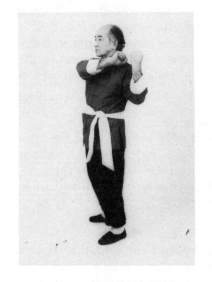

39

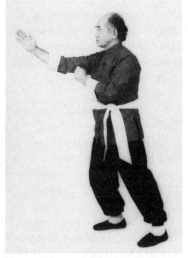

40

Sequence 13: The Tail of the Peacock

41. Cat Stance *(Mao Shih)*

Keeping your weight on your right leg, pivot on your right heel as you turn 180 degrees to your left, so that you now face East. Move your left foot with the turn of your body so that it arrives in a position to the left of your right foot. Now raise your left heel but keep the toes on the floor. As you turn, bend your left arm more and raise it so that your left fist comes in front of your left shoulder, with the front of the fist facing upwards. Your right hand should swing in a large circle with the turn of the body until it arrives underneath your left elbow, with the palm facing your body and the fingers pointing to your left (North).

42. Dragon Stance *(Lung Shih)*

Move your left foot forward a pace, then place your weight on to it as you bend your left knee and straighten your right leg. At the same time, open your left hand, slowly straighten your left arm, and push your left palm directly forward level with your shoulder. While all this is happening, turn your right palm up, and swing your right forearm outwards and upwards, then inwards and downwards, so that you have made a circle. By this time your open right hand should have arrived in the centre of your body just in front of your chest, with the palm facing downward. Now let the hand sink straight down till it arrives in front of the pelvis.

43. Monkey Stance *(Hou Shih)*

Transfer your weight on to your right leg and bend the knee slightly. Slide your left foot back so that the heel rests on the floor and the toes are raised. Circle both hands and arms forward, upward and then inwards towards your face, so that you are in a high 'on guard' position.

44. Dragon Stance *(Lung Shih)*

Rotate your wrists until your palms face forward, then slowly straighten your arms and gently push forward on a line with the shoulders. At the same time, step forward one pace with your left leg, bend your left knee, and put your weight on to your left foot, meanwhile straightening your right leg.

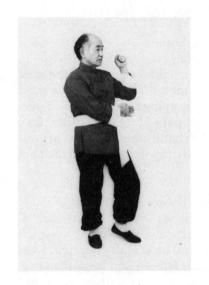

41

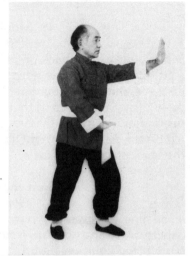

42

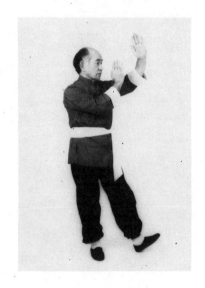

43

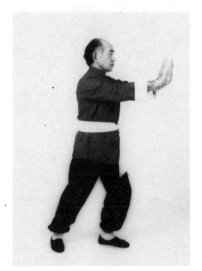

44

Sequence 14: Brush Knee and Side Step

45. Monkey Stance
(Hou Shih)

Move your weight back on to your right leg and bend the knee a little more deeply than normal. Slide your left foot back a short distance, then raise your left toes, keeping the heel on the floor. Now turn your hands so that both palms face each other, then bend your left arm so that your left hand comes in front of your left breast. Allow your right hand to drop straight down to about the level of your left knee.

46. Leopard Stance
(Pao Shih)

Turn ninety degrees to your right (South), and move your left foot forward and outward so that it is level with your right foot. Now place your weight on to your left leg and bend the knee. Rotate your wrists so that both palms face upwards, and sweep both arms upward and outward at shoulder level until the left arm is pointing directly to the left (East), and your right arm, in front of your shoulder, is pointing directly forward (South).

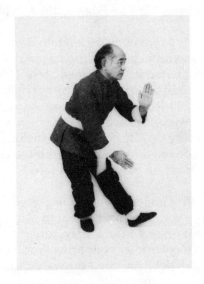

45

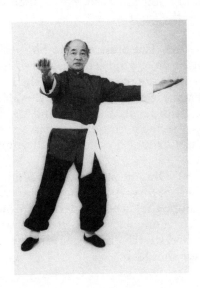

46

Sequence 15: The Edge of the Cyclone

47. Monkey Stance *(Hou Shih)*

Your right foot should step back on a diagonal line to a position to the rear of your left foot, and immediately it touches the floor put your body weight on to it and bend your right knee. Lift your left toes, but keep the left heel on the floor. As you begin to move your right foot, swing both arms upward then inwards towards your head, then very slightly downwards so that both arms cross in front of and above your forehead, with the left arm in front of your right arm. Both palms should face forward (South).

48. Dragon Stance *(Lung Shih)*

Step forward with your right foot, bending your right knee. Place your body weight on to your right leg, and straighten your left leg. As you step forward, let your arms drop all the way down in front of you, then let them circle outwards and upwards, then downwards again until they reach a position just above your right knee and about the width of your thighs apart. The fingers of both hands should point towards each other, and both palms should be facing the floor.

49. Cat Stance *(Mao Shih)*

Move your weight on to your left leg, and slide your right foot back so that the toes are in contact with the floor and the heel is raised. Move your left hand back until it is alongside your left thigh, with the palm facing the floor and the fingers pointing outwards. Slowly swing your right hand in an arc towards your left arm, so that it arrives on a level with your left elbow.

50. Dragon Stance *(Lung Shih)*

Move your right foot forward again, placing your weight on to it and bending your right knee, and at the same time straightening your left leg. In harmony with your leg movement, clench your hands into fists, and stretch your arms forward until they are on a level with your shoulders.

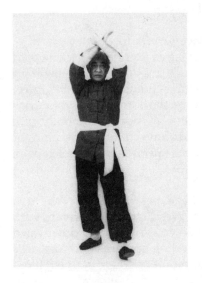

47

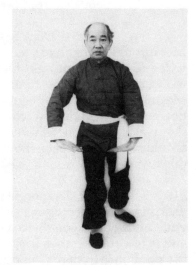

48

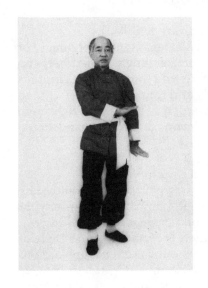

49

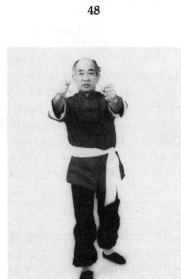

50

Sequence 16: Single Whip Unleashed

51. Duck Stance *(Ya Shih)*

Move your weight on to your left leg as you step back one pace to the rear with your right foot, placing your body weight on to it as it touches the floor, and bending your right knee. Meanwhile keep your left foot flat on the floor. Swing your arms downward, back and upwards to the right side of your body until they reach a position to the rear and above the level of your right shoulder. Your right palm should face upwards and your left palm downwards.

52. Dragon Stance *(Lung Shih)*

Turn ninety degrees to your right (West), and step forward with your left foot. As you do so, circle your right hand downward and in to your left, then keep it circling upwards and forwards to a position in front of your right shoulder. Move your left hand downwards to a point just inside your right elbow.

Sequence 17: The Double Whip

53. Cat Stance *(Mao Shih)*

Transfer your weight on to your right leg, slightly bending your right knee. Draw your left foot back, raising your left heel and keeping the left toes on the floor. As you shift your weight, turn your shoulders slightly to the left and rotate your right wrist so that your right palm faces downward, then swing your right hand to a point under your left elbow. Meanwhile your left hand should remain stationary throughout.

54. Leopard Stance *(Pao Shih)*

Step back with your left foot, bending your left knee, and bring it to a position behind your right foot. Immediately transfer your body weight on to your left leg and turn ninety degrees to your left, adjusting the angle of your left foot and then the angle of your right foot. Swing your arms outwards and upwards to shoulder level, with the palms facing outwards and the fingers pointing upwards. Now turn your head so that it looks to your left (East).

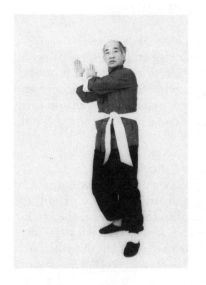

51

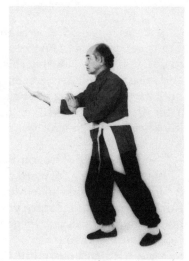

52

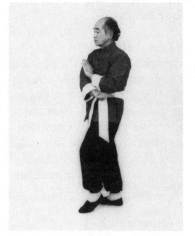

53

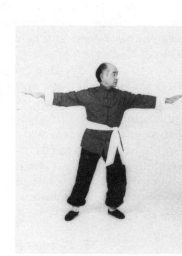

54

Sequence 18: The Playful Dog

55. Cat Stance *(Mao Shih)*

Transfer your weight on to your right leg and turn ninety degrees to your left (East). During this motion draw your left foot back and raise your left heel, keeping your left toes on the floor. Bend both arms, and swing your right arm in a big circle as you turn. Your left arm should make a smaller circle towards the right, until it arrives by the side of your right elbow.

56. Dragon Stance *(Lung Shih)*

Move your left leg forward and place your body weight on to it, whilst you bend the left knee and straighten your right leg. Rotate both wrists and turn your palms towards you, then swing both arms outwards and then inwards so that your left palm faces right (South) and your right palm faces to your left (North). Now let your left hand push directly to the right, so that your wrist and hand go beyond the right side of your right arm. Complete the circle of your right hand so that your right palm faces forward (East), then extend your right arm on a level with your shoulder, pushing with your hand. You will notice that your right arm passes over your left wrist and behind your left hand.

57. Dog Stance *(Kou Shih)*

Move your weight back on to your right leg, slightly bending the right knee. Raise your left leg forwards and up into the air, pointing the left toes directly upwards. Once the leg stops moving, drop your left toes forward. Lower your left hand, then move it to the left and upwards until it is above your left knee, with your left arm on a level with your shoulders and the left palm facing forward. Circle your right hand back, outwards and up to a position just above your right ear, with the palm facing outward.

58. Dragon Stance *(Lung Shih)*

Place your left foot on the floor, bending your left knee as you put your body weight down, and straighten your right leg. Rotate your right wrist so that the right palm faces your right cheek, and fully extend your right arm directly forward on a level with your shoulder. Your left arm should be brought back so that your left hand is alongside your right elbow.

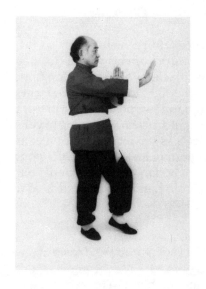

55

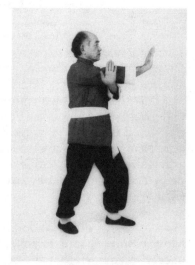

56

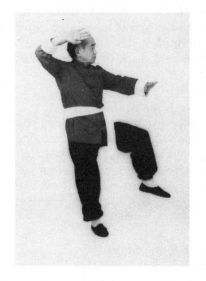

57

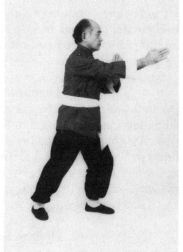

58

Sequence 19: Catching the Chickens

59. Monkey Stance *(Hou Shih)*

Turn ninety degrees to the right (South), and as you do so, step directly back with your left foot, placing your weight on to it, and bending your left knee. Slide your right foot back a few inches and raise the toes. Move your left hand to a position just in front of the right shoulder, whilst your right arm starts to swing to your right until it is over your right leg. As you start to move your right arm, rotate the wrist so that your palm faces up. Once your arm is above your leg, circle your right hand and wrist until your palm faces downwards, and drop your hand down towards your right knee.

60. Dragon Stance *(Lung Shih)*

Move your weight on to your right foot as you step forward one pace with your left foot and bend your left knee. Straighten your right leg and transfer 80% of your weight on to the left leg, and as you do this move both arms forward together. The left arm curves forward from your right shoulder to a position directly in front of your left shoulder; the right hand rotates until the palm is uppermost, while the right arm circles across the front of your body under your left arm, so that it finishes in front of your chest. At this point both hands should be extended and the fingers should be pointing forward.

61. Leopard Stance *(Pao Shih)*

A quick weight transfer is required on to your right leg as you step diagonally back and to the left with your left foot, moving your weight on to it and bending your left knee. Sweep your left hand in a curve so that it arrives in front of your right shoulder, at the same time moving the right hand outward, upward and downward in a circle until it arrives under your left arm with the palm facing your left leg.

62. Dragon Stance *(Lung Shih)*

Step forward one pace with your right leg, putting your weight on to it, and bending your right knee. Keeping your right arm slightly bent, raise it forwards and upwards in a curve until it reaches shoulder height; meanwhile the left hand drops slowly in front of the solar plexus with the fingers pointing towards your right forearm.

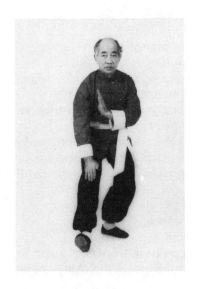

59

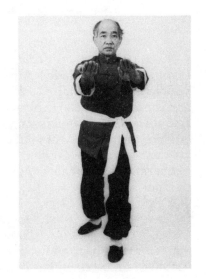

60

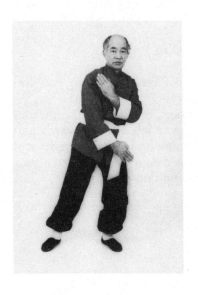

61

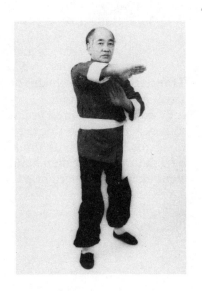

62

Sequence 20: The Archer Prepares

63. Riding Horse Stance
(Ch'i Ma Shih)

Pivoting on your right foot, turn ninety degrees to the left, taking
your left foot diagonally back and into line with your right foot,
and bending the knees deeply with your weight evenly distributed
on both legs. Meanwhile swing your arms in towards your body,
crossing them in front of your chest, then slightly upwards until
your wrists cross one another. Your left arm should be under your
right arm, your left hand by your right jaw, and your right hand
by your left jaw.

64. Dragon Stance
(Lung Shih)

Arc your right hand outwards to a point in front of your right
shoulder, almost extending the arm to its maximum. At the same
time move your right foot a pace forward and shift your body
weight on to your right leg, bending your right knee and
straightening your left leg. Gently rotate your left hand and move
it to a point just inside your right elbow.

65. Cat Stance
(Mao Shih)

Transfer your body weight on to your left leg, bending your left
knee. At the same time, slide your right foot back, and when the
foot stops moving raise your right heel, but keep your right toes
in contact with the floor. Move your left arm outwards and
forwards, pushing with your left palm, and pull your right arm
back, moving your right hand upwards to a position above your
right ear with your right palm facing outward.

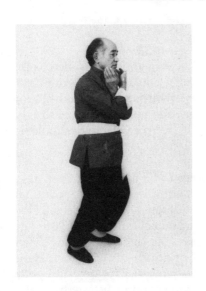

63

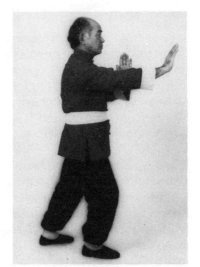

64

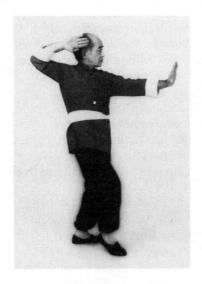

65

Sequence 21: Mount the Wild Horse

66. Dog Stance (Kou Shih)

Raise your right foot into the air, keeping your toes pulled back, but once your leg has stopped moving upwards drop your right toes forward. Curve your left arm towards yourself and stop it in front of your right chest; meanwhile your right arm slowly drops down in an arc until it is also in front of your right shoulder, and in front of your left hand.

67. Riding Horse Stance (Ch'i Ma Shih)

Turn ninety degrees to your right, swinging your right foot down on the same line as your left foot, but keeping both feet slightly more than a shoulder width apart. Correct the angle of your left foot, and bend both knees deeply. Let your right hand swing down in a curve until it is alongside your right thigh, with your right palm facing down to the floor. The left wrist rotates, and your left arm sweeps to your left, then circles round and swings back across the front of your chest until it stops in the centre line of the body, with your palm facing to the right (West).

68. Dragon Stance (Lung Shih)

Turn directly to your left so you face East once more, and then step one pace forward with your left foot, slightly diagonally to your left front. Transfer your body weight on to your left foot, bend your left knee, and straighten your right leg. As you turn, sweep your left hand outward and forward in a fairly large arc so that it finishes its movement in front of your left shoulder, fully extended, with the palm facing forward. The right hand swings to the left and upward with the movement of the body and the left hand, until it arrives on the inside of your left elbow.

69. Cat Stance (Mao Shih)

Move your body weight back on to your right leg, slightly bending the knee, at the same time sliding your left foot back towards your right foot. When the foot stops moving, raise the heel of the foot, keeping the toes on the floor. Meanwhile rotate your left wrist and circle your left hand inward, upward and slightly down, so that it ends up just above your waistline, with the palm facing the ceiling. The right hand moves back about two inches towards your chest.

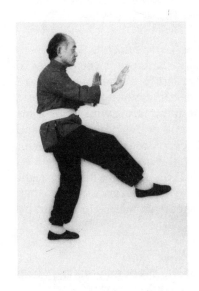

66

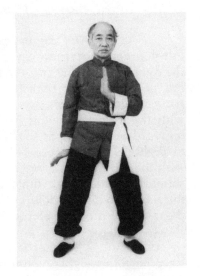

67

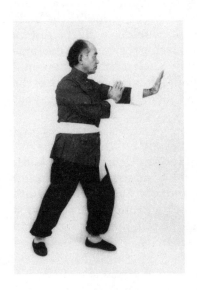

68

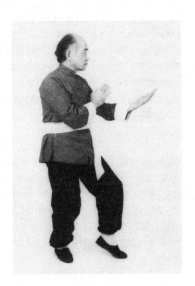

69

Sequence 22: Flexing of the Single Whip

70. Dragon Stance *(Lung Shih)*

Put your left foot firmly on the floor and pivot 180 degrees to the right. Correct the angle of your left foot, then step forward one pace with your right foot, bending your right knee and straightening your left leg. At the same time swing your arms with the motion of your body, and move your right hand outwards and forwards so that it becomes fully extended with the right palm facing forwards so that it becomes fully extended with the right palm facing forward, on a level with your right shoulder. The left wrist rotates so the left palm goes upward then turns over so it faces down, and the hand sweeps to a point by the inside of the right elbow.

71. Cat Stance *(Mao Shih)*

Keeping your weight on your right leg, pivot on your right heel as you turn 180 degrees to your left, until you once again face East. Slide your left foot back, and when it becomes stationary raise the left heel but keep your left toes on the floor. Bend your left arm upwards so the hand moves with the flow of the body until it arrives in front of your left shoulder with the fingers pointing to the ceiling and the palm facing forward. At the same time the right hand swings round in a half circular action until it reaches a point just in front of your left waist. The back of the hand faces outward and your fingers should point directly to your left (North).

72. Dragon Stance *(Lung Shih)*

Take a pace forward with your left foot and bend your left knee. Transfer your weight on to your left leg and straighten your right leg. Extend your left arm forward and rotate your left wrist until your palm faces upward; at the same time rotate your right wrist so that your right palm also faces the ceiling. Your right hand will move slightly away from your body.

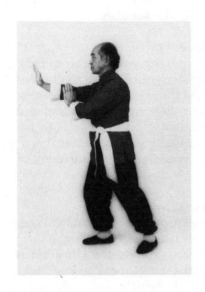

70

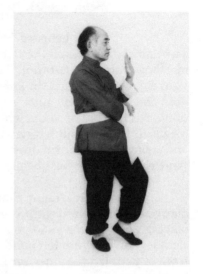

71

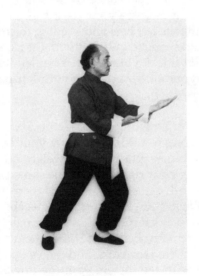

72

Sequence 23: Repulse the Monkey

73. Leopard Stance *(Pao Shih)*

Turn ninety degrees to the right, moving your right foot back
into line with your left foot. Transfer your body weight on to
your right leg and bend the knee, at the same time straightening
your left leg. As you turn, sweep your right arm round and
outwards in front of your right shoulder, with the palm facing
forward. Rotate your left wrist so that your palm faces down,
and swing your left arm down so your hand arrives in front of
your right side at waist height.

74. Dragon Stance *(Lung Shih)*

Step one pace forward with your left foot, bending your left knee,
placing your weight on to your left leg, and straightening your
right leg. Sweep your left hand directly forward to a position in
front of your left shoulder, and at the same time drop your right
hand alongside your right thigh, with the palm facing the floor.

75. Cat Stance *(Mao Shih)*

Transfer your weight on to your right leg, and draw your left
foot back, raising the left heel and keeping the toes on the floor.
Both arms should swing to your left with the right hand stopping
in front of the left side of your waist. Your left hand drops down
whilst you lift your elbow up, turn your left palm inward and
point the fingers down.

76. Dragon Stance *(Lung Shih)*

Turn ninety degrees to the left, moving your left foot forward,
bending your left knee, placing your weight on to your left leg,
and straightening your right leg. At the same time as you start
to turn, sweep both arms to your right, then swing them both
back. Your left arm straightens out and sweeps forward until it
is on a level with your left shoulder, with the palm facing forward.
Your right arm remains bent, but rotate the wrist so your hand
faces upward and then forward, and then stops in front of your
right shoulder, with the fingers pointing upwards.

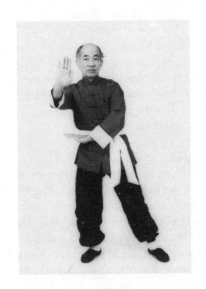

73

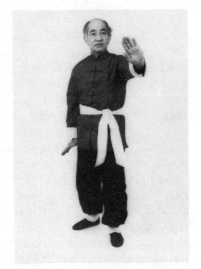

74

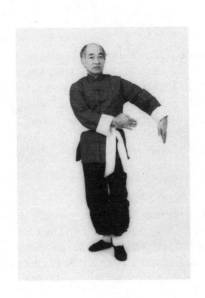

75

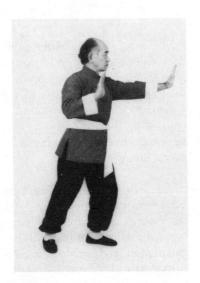

76

Sequence 24: Encompass the East and West

77. Cat Stance (*Mao Shih*)

Transfer your weight on to your right leg, and slide back your left foot. Raise the left heel, but keep the left toes on the floor. Swing your arms with a large circular motion downwards, inwards towards yourself, and up so that the palms of your hands face your chest, and your fingers point to the ceiling.

78. Dragon Stance (*Lung Shih*)

Transfer your weight on to your left leg and turn 180 degrees to your right, moving your right foot so that it comes to rest one pace ahead of your left foot. Then transfer your weight on to your right leg, bending the right knee and straightening the left leg. As you turn, sweep your right hand out and round, turning the palm outwards, until it is level with your right shoulder. Your left hand also circles with the motion of your body until it comes to rest underneath your right armpit, with the palm facing downwards.

Sequence 25: The Dog Awakens

79. Monkey Stance (*Hou Shih*)

Move your weight on to your left leg, and draw back your right foot so that you can keep your right leg straight whilst you raise your right toes. Meanwhile circle your right hand outward, upward and then downward with your little finger edge leading, until it arrives just above your right knee. Your left arm arcs upward until your left hand is just above your left ear, with the palm facing outward.

80. Dog Stance (*Kou Shih*)

Raise your right leg into the air, pointing the toes upwards to the ceiling, and when the leg is in its new position drop the toes forward. Circle your right arm to the left and upwards, bending the arm in front of your right shoulder, and your left hand arcs outward and downward until it is alongside your left thigh, with the palm facing the floor.

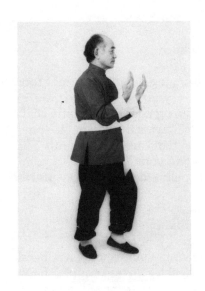

77

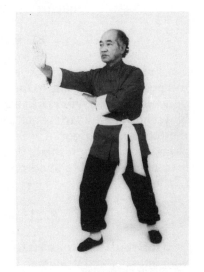

78

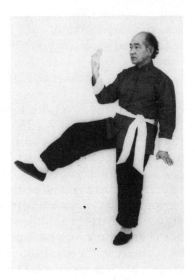

79

80

Sequence 26: Roll and Stretch

81. Cat Stance
(Mao Shih)

Turn ninety degrees to the left, bringing down your right foot
to a position behind and to the right of your left foot, and transfer
your weight on to your right leg, keeping your knee slightly bent.
Now slide your left foot back a little, raising the heel but keeping
the toes on the floor. Circle your right arm down until it is
alongside your right thigh, and swing your left hand to a point
in front of your right shoulder. Both palms should face downwards
to the floor.

82. Dragon Stance
(Lung Shih)

Step forward with your left foot and put your weight on it, bend
your left knee and straighten your right leg. Sweep your left hand
forwards in an arc to a position directly in front of, and in line
with, your left shoulder. Let your right hand lightly swing forward
in front of your body, then let it rise up under your right elbow
with the palm naturally facing up towards the ceiling, then let
it sweep forward under your left arm until it is alongside your
left arm and hand. All your fingers should point directly forward.

Sequence 27: The Five Elements

83. Riding Horse Stance
(Ch'i Ma Shih)

Rotate your right wrist so that your right hand sweeps down
towards your body, then turn it over and slightly up, then outward
past the width of your body. Now turn your fingers so that they
point to the ceiling, and bring your arm towards the centre line
of your body. Your left arm meanwhile bends, and is slowly
drawn towards the middle of your body, so that the palms of
both hands now face each other. At the same time, turn forty-
five degrees to the left (East) moving your left foot back beyond
your right foot, and pivoting on your right heel. Your feet should
now be a little wider than the width of your shoulders apart and
both knees should be bent.

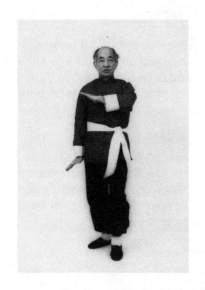

81

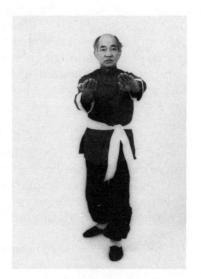

82

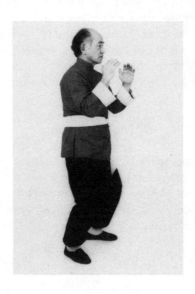

83

84. Dragon Stance
(Lung Shih)

Step forward one pace with the left foot, putting your weight on to it as you bend the left knee, and straighten the right leg. Then curve your hands inward, upward and forward so that the palms face up, and the fingers of both hands point forward, with both arms extended.

85. Cat Stance
(Mao Shih)

Move your left foot back a little, raising the heel and keeping the toes on the floor. Rotate your hands outward, inwards and downwards, so that your palms face down and the tips of your fingers are the width of your thighs apart.

86. Leopard Stance
(Pao Shih)

Step forward about twelve inches with your left foot, and before your weight is fully on it, turn your left toes to the right, pivoting on your left heel. Turn your body ninety degrees to the right, and correct the angle of your right foot. Bend your left knee, and straighten your right leg. Simultaneously, swing your left hand up to a position in front of your right shoulder, whilst your right hand rotates, palm up, then swings to the right and sweeps back to a position under your left elbow, with the palm facing your left thigh.

87. Monkey Stance
(Hou Shih)

Turn ninety degrees to the right (West), keeping your body weight on your left leg, draw back your right foot and raise your right toes. Circle your right arm upwards until the palm is in front of your right shoulder, with the palm facing inward. Your left hand moves slightly downwards, with the palm down.

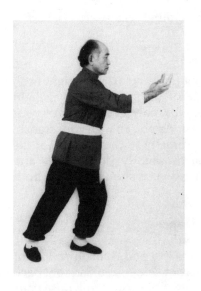

84

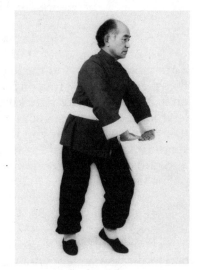

85

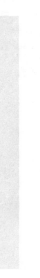

86

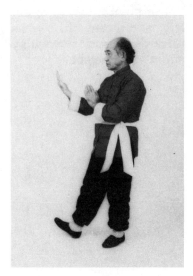

87

Sequence 28: The Double Whip

88. Leopard Stance
(Pao Shih)

Turn your right toes to the left by pivoting on your right heel, then place your right foot on the floor and put your body weight on to it, bending your right knee. Now correct the angle of your left foot and straighten your left leg. As you change your stance, turn your head so that you look directly to the left, and at the same time sweep both your arms slightly downwards and outwards until they are in line with your shoulders with both palms facing down.

89. Cat Stance
(Mao Shih)

Turn your body ninety degrees to the left, and pivot on your right heel to alter the angle of your right foot. Move your left foot back a little, then keep your left toes on the floor whilst you raise your left heel. As your body is turning draw both arms towards the centre line of your body, bending your left arm so that your left fingers point to the ceiling and your palm faces to the right. Your left hand meanwhile swings across the body, so that it faces towards your left side with your left arm close to your body at about waist height.

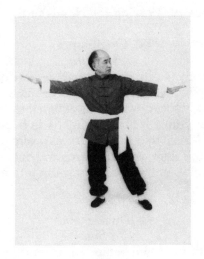

88

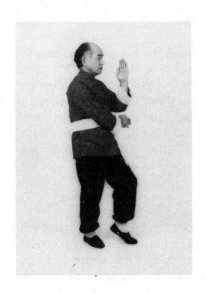

89

Sequence 29: Waving the Hands in the Clouds

90. Dog Stance
(Kou Shih)

Keeping your body weight on your right leg, swing your left foot forwards and upwards with the toes raised, and when the leg stops moving point your toes down. Raise your left elbow and forearm upwards so that your left hand is slightly in front of and above your forehead. Meanwhile turn your right palm up as you sweep your hand to your right, then upwards and downwards, so that it moves down the centre line of your body to a point in front of the abdomen.

91. Duck Stance
(Ya Shih)

Swing your left foot down behind your right foot to the floor, bending your left knee, and slide your right foot back slightly while keeping it flat on the floor. Move your left hand back to just above your left ear, and move your right hand a little further forward, palm down.

92. Dragon Stance
(Lung Shih)

Move your left leg one pace forward ahead of your right foot, left knee bent, and place your body weight on to it whilst the right leg straightens. Push your left palm directly forward in line with your left shoulder, and swing your right arm across your chest, finishing with the right hand, palm down, close to your left side.

93. Snake Stance
(She Shih)

Draw your left foot back slightly so that your body weight is evenly distributed on both legs. Swing your right arm down, then backwards and up, so that it is vertical, the palm facing to your left. Your left hand follows the swing of your right arm by moving across your body to a point underneath your right armpit, with the fingers pointing upwards.

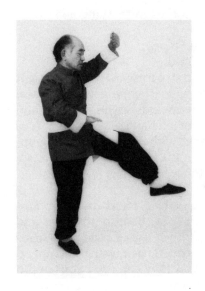

90

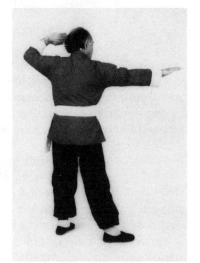

91

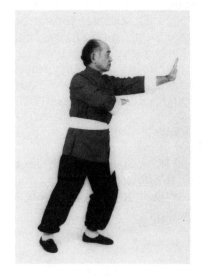

92

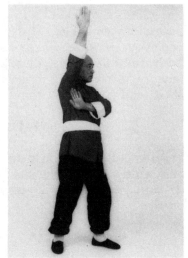

93

Sequence 30: Consoling the North Wind

94. Dragon Stance
(Lung Shih)

Turn ninety degrees to the right and step forward with your right foot, transferring your weight on to it and bending the right knee. Swing your right arm outward, downwards, then slightly up and forwards in front of your chest. Your left hand rotates and sweeps across the centre line of your body, with both palms facing up.

95. Riding Horse Stance
(Ch'i Ma Shih)

Move your body weight on to your left leg, then bring your right foot back into line with your left foot. Bend both knees and distribute your weight evenly on both legs. Circle your arms upwards above the height of your head, then outwards and down, then slightly up and inwards so that they end up, palms up, in front of the centre line of your waist.

96. Dragon Stance
(Lung Shih)

Put your body weight on to your right leg, and step forward a pace with your left leg. Then put your weight on the left leg and bend your left knee, while you straighten your right leg. Sweep both arms forward as you rotate your wrists so that the palms face down. Your left arm should end up bowed in front of your chest, and your right behind it, roughly forming a letter 't'.

97. Duck Stance
(Ya Shih)

Transfer your weight on to your right leg, and slide your left foot back a little, keeping the foot flat on the floor. Swing both arms down and then up over your right shoulder, keeping both palms open.

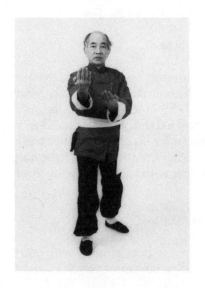

94

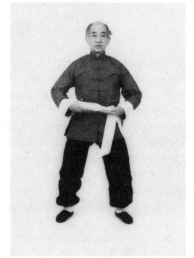

95

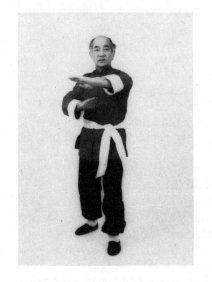

96

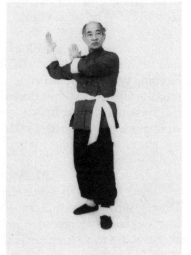

97

Sequence 31: The Leopard Shows its Teeth

98. Dragon Stance
(Lung Shih)

Turn ninety degrees to the right, moving your weight on to your left leg whilst stepping forward with your right foot, bending your right knee. Then transfer your weight on to your right leg, and straighten your left leg. Sweep and extend your left hand to a position in front of your left shoulder, with the palm facing forward. Your right hand moves with the natural swing to a point in front of the left side of your chest, with the palm facing your left biceps.

99. Leopard Stance
(Pao Shih)

Turn ninety degrees to the left, stepping back slightly with your left foot, bending your left knee and placing most of your weight on to that leg. Straighten your right leg. As you turn, bend your left arm, turn the right palm up, and swing your right hand outwards, upwards then inwards again, with both hands parallel to each other and the fingers pointing upwards. Your hands should stop in front of your chest.

100. Dog Stance
(Kou Shih)

Keeping your weight on your left leg, swing your right leg forward into the air with the toes raised; when the foot stops moving drop the toes down. Your hands, meanwhile, should move sideways, still parallel to each other, until your right hand is in front of your left shoulder.

101. Monkey Stance
(Hou Shih)

Drop your right foot down to the rear of your left foot, whilst turning ninety degrees to your left (East). Slide your left foot back slightly and raise the toes. Turn your right palm towards your chest, and swing your left arm downwards and across in front of your abdomen, then upwards until both arms are crossed in front of the chest.

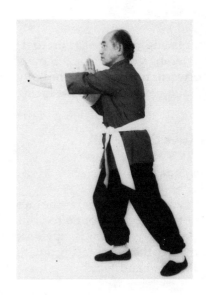

98

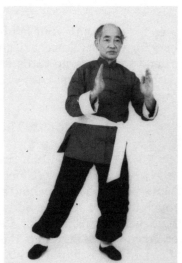

99

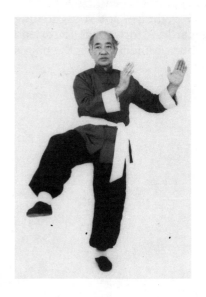

100

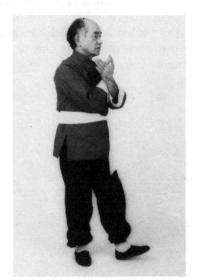

101

102. Dragon Stance
(Lung Shih)

Step forward with your left foot, placing your weight on to it, bending your left knee, and straightening your right leg. Slowly extend your arms, upwards and forwards to the front of the body with the hands level with your shoulders and the palms facing towards you.

Sequence 32: The Scissors Cut the Silk

103. Scissor Stance
(Chien Tao Shih)

Move your right foot behind and beyond your left leg; as the toes touch the floor spin the body about 110 degrees round to your right, with both knees bent. Circle both arms outwards, upwards and downwards in front of the body with the palms facing down; the right hand should be above the left hand.

104. Dragon Stance
(Lung Shih)

Step forward one pace with your right foot, bending your right knee, placing your weight on your right leg, and straightening your left leg. Move both hands upward and forward as you extend your arms directly in line with your shoulders, with the palms facing the ceiling.

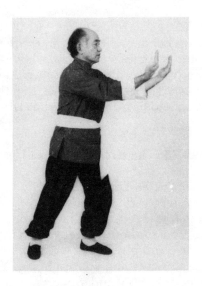

102

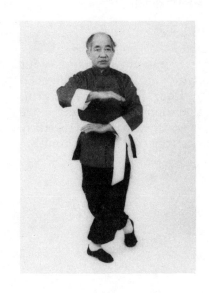

103

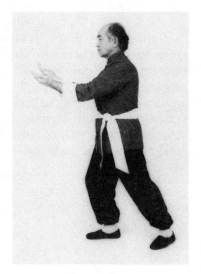

104

105. Crane Stance
(Hao Shih)

Raise your left leg, bending the knee, and with the toes raised. As soon as the leg becomes stationary, allow the toes to drop down. Rotate both wrists so the palms face down, then sweep both arms sideways. The right only moves slightly to your right, but the left arm should be extended to your left on a level with your shoulder.

Sequence 33: The Archer Releases His Arrow

106. Dragon Stance
(Lung Shih)

Turn 180 degrees to the left, pivoting on your right foot, and lowering your left foot to about a pace away from your right foot. Bend your left knee and place your weight on to your left leg, at the same time straightening your right leg. Your right hand should move over your head and forwards on a level with your forehead. Your left hand, meanwhile, is drawn in a half circular action to a position in front of your solar plexus.

107. Cat Stance
(Mao Shih)

Draw back your left foot as you transfer your weight on to your right leg. When your left foot stops moving, raise your left heel, keeping the toes in contact with the floor. Bend your right arm, and draw your right hand back to a position just behind and above your right ear, with the index finger and thumb pressed together. Your left hand is pushed forward in front of your left shoulder, with the palm facing away.

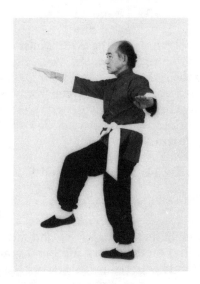

105

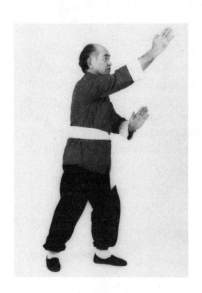

106

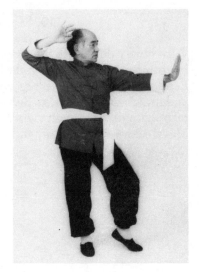

107

108. Dragon Stance
(Lung Shih)

Place your left foot firmly on the floor whilst you step forward one pace with your right foot. As your right foot becomes implanted bend the right knee, place your weight on your right leg, and straighten your left leg. Sweep your right hand to the left in front of your chest, then forward with palm turned upwards. Your left hand should swing down beside your left thigh, with the palm facing down.

Sequence 34: Brush Knee and Side Step

109. Duck Stance
(Ya Shih)

Transfer your weight on to your left leg and slide your right foot back, keeping it flat on the floor, and bend your left knee and body forward. Rotate your right wrist so your hand goes outward and downward, arriving just above your right knee with the palm down. Your left hand, meanwhile, is brought up to a position in front of your chest, with the palm facing to your right.

110. Leopard Stance
(Pao Shih)

Turn ninety degrees to the right (South), and then step sideways to your right so that your right foot is in line with your left foot. Bend your right knee, place your weight on to your right leg, and straighten your left leg. Sweep both hands to your right, palms facing down, until your right hand is extended to your right on a level with your shoulder, and your left hand is by your right side.

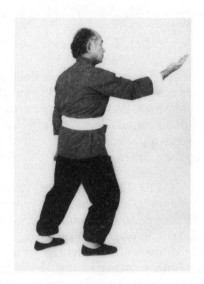

108

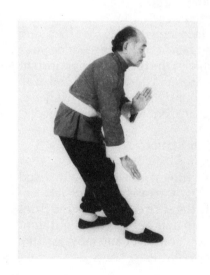

109

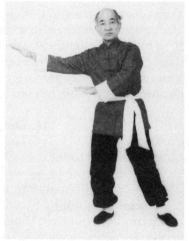

110

Sequence 35: Within the Cyclone

111. Cat Stance
(Mao Shih)

Place your weight on to your left leg, knee bent, whilst you turn ninety degrees to your right (West). Slide your right foot back, then raise your right heel. Bend your right arm and then circle both hands inwards and upwards in front of your body until your fingers point upwards and your palms face your chest with your hands parallel to each other.

112. Dragon Stance
(Lung Shih)

Move your right foot forward, bending your right knee and placing your weight on to your right leg. Straighten your left leg. Circle both hands outwards, slightly upwards, and then downwards until both wrists cross just above your right knee, with your right wrist on the top. Both palms should face down.

113. Monkey Stance
(Hou Shih)

Turn ninety degrees to the left, moving your left foot back and placing your weight on to it, and bend the left knee. Slide your right foot back slightly and then raise the toes. Circle your right hand out to your right, then upwards and down so that you drop it above and slightly inwards of your right knee. Your left hand, meanwhile, moves up to a position in front of your right shoulder.

114. Dragon Stance
(Lung Shih)

Move your right foot forward, shifting your weight on to it and bending your right knee, whilst you straighten your left leg. Clench your right hand into a fist and circle it across the front of your body to your left, then up and out to your right until it is in front of your right shoulder. Your left hand moves a little further forward inside your right elbow.

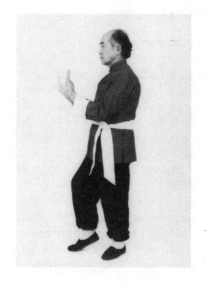

111

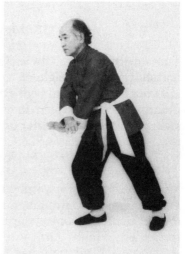

112

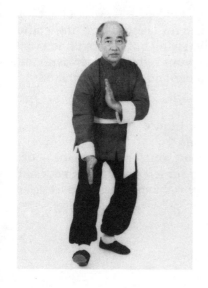

113

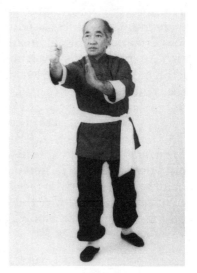

114

Sequence 36: The Wild Horse Resists

115. Monkey Stance
(Hou Shih)

Turn ninety degrees to the left, stepping back with your right foot, and shifting your weight on to it. Raise the toes of your left foot. Lift your left hand until your arm is perpendicular, with the fingers pointing up and the palm facing right. Your clenched right hand swings with the turn of the body to a point under your left elbow.

116. Dragon Stance
(Lung Shih)

Move your left leg forward, putting your weight on to it, bending your left knee and straightening the right leg. Swing both hands to your right, then open your right hand as you sweep both hands to the left. The left arm extends until it is in front of the left shoulder, and the right hand finishes inside your left elbow.

117. Crane Stance
(Hao Shih)

Transfer your weight on to your right leg, and lift your left leg up in the air with toes raised. When the leg stops moving let the toes drop down. Simultaneously, swing both arms up to your right, so both hands finish above your right shoulder, with the left hand in front of the left shoulder and the right hand out to the right.

118. Leopard Stance
(Pao Shih)

Turn ninety degrees to the right, place your left foot on the floor, put your weight on it, and bend your left knee. Turn your left hand so that your palm faces your right shoulder, and let your right hand swing down and up in a big arc until it stops just underneath your left elbow.

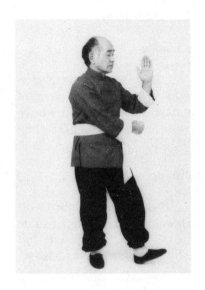

115

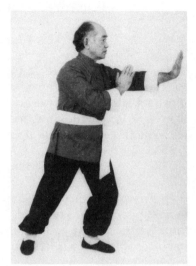

116

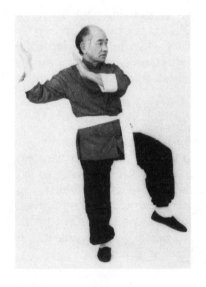

117

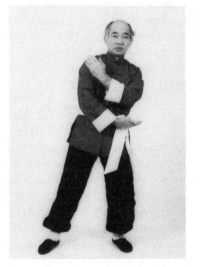

118

Sequence 37: The Playful Monkey

119. Monkey Stance
(Hou Shih)

Move your weight on to your right leg, stepping back with your left foot and transferring your weight on to it. Slide your right foot back slightly, then raise the toes. Swing both arms outwards, then circle your hands inwards to a position in front of your chest with the fingers pointing up.

120. Dragon Stance
(Lung Shih)

Step forward with your right leg and put your weight on it, bending your right knee and straightening your left leg. Rotate your wrists so that your palms face outward. Sweep your left hand directly to your left, and push your right hand forward, extending both arms.

121. Duck Stance
(Ya Shih)

Transfer your weight on to your left leg, allowing your right foot to slide back a little with the foot flat on the floor. Circle your left arm inwards towards your body, then upwards until the fingers point to the ceiling. Your right hand sweeps back across the front of your body until your hand stops near your left armpit with the palm facing down.

122. Dragon Stance
(Lung Shih)

Transfer your weight on to your right leg and turn ninety degrees to the left (East). Now step forward with your left foot, placing your weight on to it, and bending your left knee whilst you straighten your right leg. Circle your left hand to the right, then sweep it directly forward, extending it as it comes level with your left shoulder. Your right hand drops gently downwards until it reaches your waistline, palm still facing down.

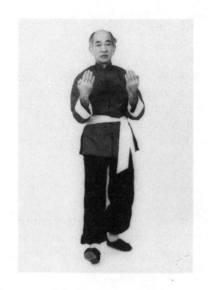

119

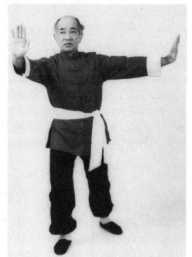

120

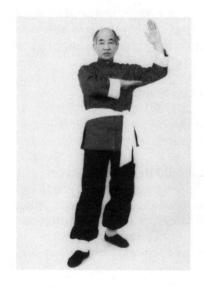

121

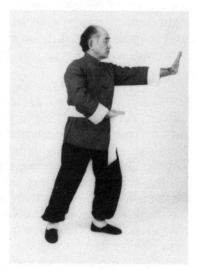

122

Sequence 38: The Chickens Become Excited

123. Duck Stance
(Ya Shih)
Draw your body weight back on to your right leg, and as you do so, slide your left foot back a little, keeping it flat on the floor. Circle your left hand clockwise to about hip height with the palm facing down. At the same time circle your right arm upwards and back, so that your right hand stops above your right ear, with the palm facing outward.

124. Dog Stance
(Kou Shih)
Keeping your weight on your right leg, raise your left leg into the air. As you do so, circle both arms downwards, inwards towards the centre line of your body, then upwards and outwards, with both palms facing upwards.

125. Monkey Stance
(Hou Shih)
Swing your left foot down to the floor, slightly ahead of your right foot, then raise your left toes. Circle your arms upwards and inwards and slightly down until they cross in front of your forehead, with the right arm in front of the left arm.

126. Crossed Leg Stance
(P'anche T'ui Shih)
Lower your left toes, and as you do so pivot on your left heel, turning your body ninety degrees to the right (South). Now step sideways to your left with your right foot, crossing in front of your left leg. Your body weight should be maintained on your left leg, and your right toes should only lightly touch the floor. Now swing both arms down the centre line of the body, then outwards and upwards until both arms are on a level with your shoulders with your palms facing outward.
(The photograph for this stance has been taken a fraction late, and shows the weight changing to move into the next stance).

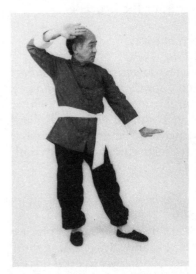

123

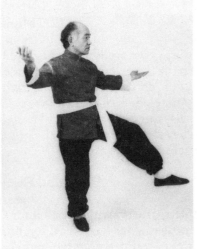

124

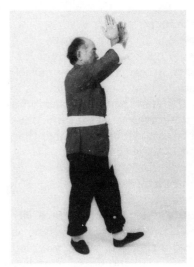

125

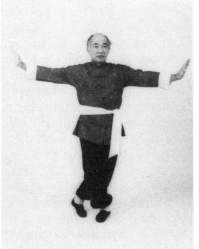

126

Sequence 39: Eight Strands of the Brocade

127. Monkey Stance
(Hou Shih)

Place your weight on your right leg by lowering your right heel
to the floor. Turn ninety degrees to your right (West), swinging
your left foot behind your right and bringing it to rest behind
your right foot. Now place your weight on to your left leg and
raise the toes of your right foot. Move both hands inward so that
they stop at about waist height, parallel to each other, with both
palms facing inwards.

128. Dragon Stance
(Lung Shih)

Step forward with your left foot, bending your left knee, placing
most of your weight on to your left leg and straightening your
right leg. Push your left hand forward and upward until it is on
a line with your left shoulder, with the palm facing forward. Turn
your right hand in a small circle so that your right palm ends up
in front of your abdomen.

129. Cat Stance
(Mao Shih)

Turn ninety degrees to the left, step back with your right foot
and place your weight on to your right leg. Now slide your left
foot back a little, raising your left heel but keeping the toes in
contact with the floor. Sweep your left hand round towards your
right armpit with the palm facing downwards. At the same time,
swing your right hand upwards so that it is slightly higher than
your right shoulder, with the palm facing forward.

130. Dragon Stance
(Lung Shih)

Turn ninety degrees to the left (East) and step forward a pace with
your left foot, bending your left knee, placing your weight on
to your left leg, and straightening your right leg. Swing your left
hand round to a point in front of your left shoulder, extending
it forward as it moves. Your right hand sweeps across the front
of your body until it arrives near your left armpit, with the palm
facing down.

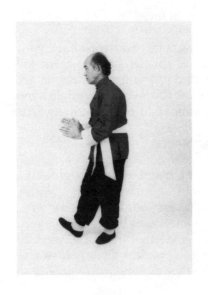

127

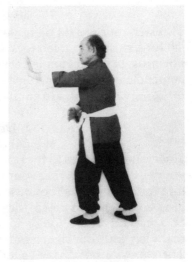

128

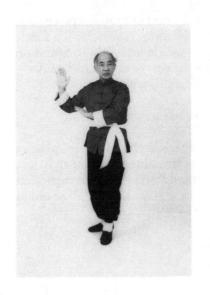

129

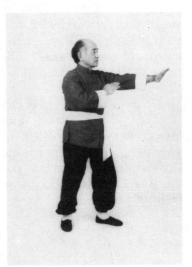

130

131. Monkey Stance
(Hou Shih)

Transfer your weight on to your right leg, and draw back your left foot, raising your left toes. Circle your left hand inwards and upwards, bending your left arm, and stop when your fingers are perpendicular and your palm faces towards you. Your right hand makes a very small arc so that your right palm faces inward.

132. Dog Stance
(Kou Shih)

Lower your left toes to the floor and transfer your weight on to your left leg, then swing your right foot forwards and upwards into the air with the toes raised. When your leg stops moving, drop your right toes down. Meanwhile, swing both arms outward on a line with your shoulders, with the left arm pointing directly to the left and your right hand fingers pointing directly forward. The palms of both hands should face downwards.

133. Monkey Stance
(Hou Shih)

Swing your right foot down behind your left foot and place your weight on to your right leg, raising the toes of your left foot. Circle both arms outwards, upwards and then downwards, to a position in front of your left knee, with the fingers of each hand pointing to each other and the palms pressing downwards.

134. Dragon Stance
(Lung Shih)

Step forward with the left foot, bending the left knee, placing your weight on to your left leg, and straightening your right leg. Rotate your wrists so that your hands circle inwards, upwards and then forwards, and, palms outward, push your arms out in front of you.

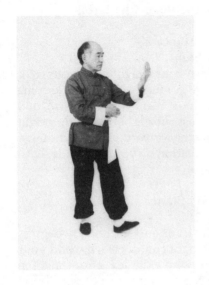

131

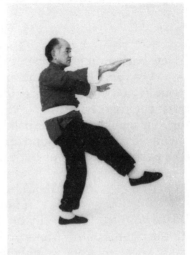

132

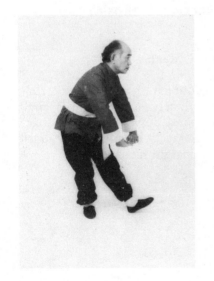

133

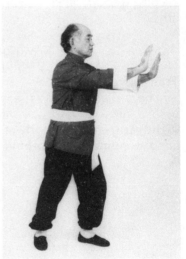

134

Sequence 40: Enclose the Inner Ch'i Orbit

135. Cat Stance
(Mao Shih)

Draw back your left foot and place your weight on to your right leg. When your left foot stops moving, raise your left heel, keeping your left toes in contact with the floor. Bend your right arm, and raise your right hand to a position just outside but above the height of your shoulder, with the palm facing forward. At the same time, swing your left hand round to a position by your right side, with the palm towards your body.

136. Dragon Stance
(Lung Shih)

Place your left foot firmly on the floor and turn ninety degrees to the right (South). Move your right foot forward, bend your right knee, put your weight on to your right leg, and straighten your left leg. Bring your hands to the centre line of your body and rotate the wrists so your hands circle downwards towards each other, then upwards and downwards again in a small circle, keeping them parallel to each other with both palms facing each other.

137. Monkey Stance
(Hou Shih)

Transfer your weight back on to your left leg and slide your right foot back slightly, then raise your right toes. As you do so, circle both hands outwards, upwards and downwards, then back slightly towards your body at about waist height, with your left hand stopping a little behind your right hand.

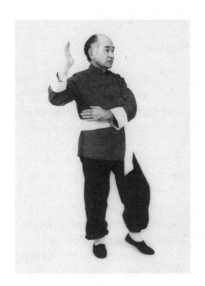

135

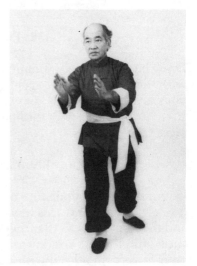

136

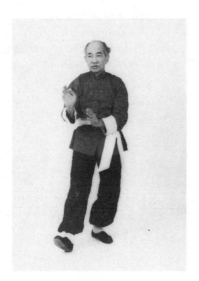

137

Sequence 41: Gather Earth's Energy

138. Eagle Stance
(Ying Shih)

Draw back your right foot until it rests alongside your left foot with your body weight evenly distributed on both legs. Circle your arms downwards, upwards and outwards until they are stretched out level with the line of the shoulders, with the palms facing outwards.

139. Eagle Stance
(Ying Shih)

Without moving your feet or your weight, swing your arms downwards and inwards towards the centre line of your body, and then upwards so that they end up crossed in front of your chest with the left arm in front of the right arm and the tips of your fingers on a level with your shoulders.

Sequence 42: Finish

140. Eagle Stance
(Ying Shih)

Allow your arms to swing down slowly so that they come to rest alongside your thighs.

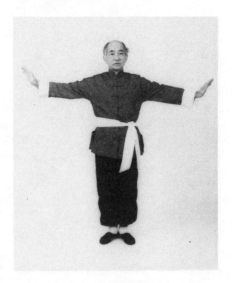

138

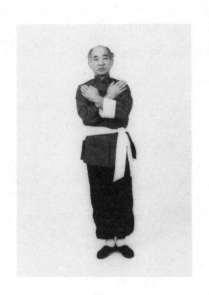

139

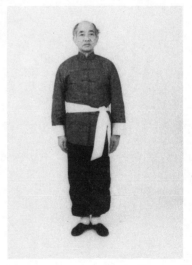

140

Chapter 13

The Benefits of T'ai Chi Ch'uan

In many photographs and films of T'ai Chi being performed, the performers shown are generally older people. As a result many people have the impression that T'ai Chi is not for the young. This is quite wrong, for ideally a person should practise the art from early childhood onwards, so as to enjoy the best of health for as long as possible. T'ai Chi is an ancient form of therapeutic exercise which can be practised by young and old alike.

The gentleness of T'ai Chi ensures that anyone practising it does not suffer strains and other muscular injuries, but obtains greater strength while developing greater flexibility and suppleness. Dedicated athletes will find that T'ai Chi is one of the finest possible ways of gently warming up, and helps to offset any vigorous exercise that may follow. For a person practising T'ai Chi, sleep is deep and restful, and the nervous system will be soothed and calmed, so as to ensure tranquillity at all times. Those who suffer from certain forms of illness, such as arthritis, rheumatism, lumbago, sciatica or multiple sclerosis, can receive great benefit from practising T'ai Chi, as can anyone suffering from weight problems, for the exercise helps to break down the fat tissue, thereby reducing the body weight to its natural level.

Another of the great benefits from T'ai Chi is the way it sharpens the mental faculties, so that a very strong and purposeful mind is developed. Dynamic and exact control is maintained over all parts of the body, and by this means one also learns to keep control of one's emotions, and to develop a deep inner peace, thereby becoming at one with oneself and with others around you. This naturally leads to a greater awareness and understanding of oneself, and a greater appreciation and understanding of others. All this creates wonderful harmony within ourselves, and with the world around us.

Added to this, one becomes much more vital, learning to use one's energies to the full. A person who practises T'ai Chi develops the ability to work for long hours without suffering the slightest sign of strain, and eventually has so much energy that they can give some of it to others in many different ways. Constant practise of T'ai Chi also aids the development of mental and spiritual energies, thereby opening up the vast field of Taoist Meditation.

Thus there are enormous benefits to be gained from the practise of T'ai Chi Ch'uan. If you take it up and practise regularly and with dedication, you will soon find that your life is taking on a new meaning, and that you are becoming more positive and purposeful. Having started, keep on, for there is no end to the road in front of you.

When strains are no longer felt, strains disappear.
When stresses are not experienced, stresses vanish.
When aggression is not recognized, it does not exist.
When badness is not seen, it ceases to be prevalent.

When we no longer think of goodness, it disappears.
When we do not think of hate and evil, they both vanish.
When we do not recognize 'I', it does not exist.
When earth is not seen, then earth ceases to be prevalent.

When we no longer compare one with another, then all disappear, and we understand the Tao.

International Taoist Society

You may be interested to know that this Society is based on the foundations that were originally laid down by Professor Chan Kam Lee, who started the first Chinese Taoist Arts School in London in 1930.

Chan Lee died in the winter of 1953-4, when his boat sank in a fierce storm off the coast of China, and it was then that his nephew Chee Soo was asked to take over the Presidency of all the Taoist Arts that were being taught. In 1958, Chee Soo set up coaching classes with the object of training qualified teachers, and county, area and regional coaches. Over the years these have proved very successful and there are now classes and clubs operating in many parts of the world, besides those that exist in the British Isles.

Our Society only teaches the Taoist arts of 'The Eight Strands of the Brocade', which comprise:

Ch'ang Ming	—	Taoist Long Life Dietary Health Therapy
Ts'ao Yao	—	Taoist Herbal Therapy
An Mo	—	Taoist Massage
Tao Yin	—	Taoist Respiration Therapy
Tien Chen	—	Taoist Spot Pressing (Acupressure)
Chili Nung	—	Ch'i, Li, Vibration and Palm Healing
Chen Tuan	—	Taoist Diagnosis Techniques

There are two associations who are federated members of our Society, The Chinese Cultural Arts Association, who teach:

T'ai Chi Ch'uan	—	The Supreme Ultimate
K'ai Men	—	Taoist Yoga (Chi Kung)
I Fu Shou	—	Sticky or Adhering Hands
Li Kung	—	Taoist development of Li energy
Mo Kun	—	Taoist Wand — external energy control
Mo Hsiang	—	Taoist Meditation

Also T'ai Chi Sword, T'ai Chi Sabre, T'ai Chi Stick and T'ai Chi Dance.

and The International Wu Shu Association, who teach:

Feng Shou	—	'Hand of the Wind Kungfu, soft and gentle but very fast, and suitable for all age groups.
Chi Shu	—	Taoist form of Aikido

and all the other forms of the Taoist fighting arts including such weapons as sticks, flails, swords and chopsticks.

Needless to say, all three associations work together, and all strictly maintain the traditions that were laid down by Chan Kam Lee and his family.

Our President, Chee Soo, is naturally also a Taoist, and his whole life is dedicated to serving the sick and suffering, and to helping humanity whenever possible.

Anyone who is interested in any of these arts can attend the student classes which are held regularly in the British Isles and on the Continent. Weekend courses are also held, together with workshops at Easter and Christmas and in the summer. Please write for further information to:

The International Taoist Society
426 Charter Avenue
Canley
Coventry CV4 8BD
West Midlands
England

Index